Passing the FRCPath
Part 1 Examination:

A Practical
Guide for
Haematology
Registrars

Passing the FRCPath
Part 1 Examination:
A Practical
Guide for
Haematology
Registrars

Dr Joel McCay

Haematology Specialist Registrar, London, UK

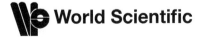 **World Scientific**

NEW JERSEY · LONDON · SINGAPORE · BEIJING · SHANGHAI · HONG KONG · TAIPEI · CHENNAI · TOKYO

Published by

World Scientific Publishing Co. Pte. Ltd.

5 Toh Tuck Link, Singapore 596224

USA office: 27 Warren Street, Suite 401-402, Hackensack, NJ 07601

UK office: 57 Shelton Street, Covent Garden, London WC2H 9HE

Library of Congress Control Number: 2024935426

British Library Cataloguing-in-Publication Data
A catalogue record for this book is available from the British Library.

PASSING THE FRCPATH PART 1 EXAMINATION
A Practical Guide for Haematology Registrars

ISBN 978-981-12-8020-7 (hardcover)
ISBN 978-981-12-8021-4 (ebook for institutions)
ISBN 978-981-12-8022-1 (ebook for individuals)

For any available supplementary material, please visit
https://www.worldscientific.com/worldscibooks/10.1142/13514#t=suppl

About the author

Joel is a haematology registrar working primarily in Northwest London but currently in research at Barts Cancer Institute. He graduated from the University of Southampton in 2014 before undertaking foundation training in Northeast England, core medical training in Southeast London before securing his haematology registrar number in 2019. He sat the FRCPath Part 1 exam in 2020 and realised that a shorthand revision guide compiling the guidelines was missing. The following handbook addresses that problem and is also a helpful go-to while on the ward. He has worked with start-up bio-tech companies, the British Medical Journal as an editor for their revision resource as well as working alongside some of the leading haematology doctors in the country at The London Clinic. His research is in CLL subtypes and the role non-coding RNA from extracellular vesicles impacts the cells of the tumour microenvironment. Joel is a keen runner, father to his daughter Daphne and enthusiastic Liverpool Football Club fan.

Dedicated to Nancy Thomas, the only teacher to believe in me when I first said I wanted to be a doctor. To my parents, Sharon and Robert, for all the endless support they have given me over the years and for always being kind. To my wife, Charlie, for being understanding, caring and compassionate, without whom I would not be able to be the person I am. And to my daughter Daphne, who brings me endless joy.

Editors and reviewers

Red Cell Haematology:
Dr Mamta Sohal MRCP FRCPath. Consultant haematologist. Hammersmith hospital, Imperial Healthcare NHS trust

Haematological Oncology:
Professor John G Gribben MD DSc FRCP FRCPath, FHEA, FMedSci
Hamilton Fairley Chair of Medical Oncology, Barts Cancer Institute, Queen Mary University of London
Honorary Consultant in Haemato-Oncology, St Bartholomew's Hospital, London

Dr Akila Danga MBBS BSC FRCPath. Consultant haematologist. The Hillingdon hospital NHS Foundation trust

Transfusion:
Dr Richard Kaczmarski MBBS MD FRCP FRCPath. Consultant haematologist. The Hillingdon hospital NHS Foundation trust

Haemostasis and Thrombosis:
Dr Carolyn Millar MD Med FRCP FRCPath. Consultant haematologist and clinical senior lecturer. Hammersmith hospital, Imperial Healthcare NHS trust

Content editing and revisions:
Mr Charlie Butler

Artwork and design:
Mrs Becky Mitchell

Foreword

What attracted most of us to a career in haematology was the blend of laboratory and clinical medicine, spread across areas as diverse as transfusion, red cell, haematological oncology and haemostasis and thrombosis. Possession of both MRCP and FRCPath is a mandatory requirement for you to be awarded your CCT in haematology. Not all specialities have an "exit examination" but haematology is one that does. The FRCPath examination is designed to assess your knowledge, skill and behaviour in the fields detailed in the haematology curriculum and is a rite of passage for all Haematology trainees. Therein lies your first problem, as the topics to cover in the haematology curriculum for the exam encompass the whole scope of the diverse fields of laboratory and clinical haematology.

Part 1 of the FRCPath examination comprises 2 written papers evaluating your knowledge and clinical judgement. The part 1 examination is used to determine whether you have attained an acceptable level of knowledge and reached an acceptable level of competence based on the objectives of the training programme. You must achieve a pass mark in both papers at a single sitting to pass the part 1 examination.

Paper 1 lasts 3 hours and comprises 4 compulsory essay questions. You must answer all 4 questions and preach an acceptable mark in each, remembering not to spend too much time on any a particular essay that you may know much more about. It is significantly harder to gain additional marks in any question than to get the pass you need from the basics of each of the 4 essay questions. The questions address important areas of the 4 domains mentioned already and largely cover both laboratory and/or clinical practice in each. The essay questions are designed to explore your abilities to communicate effectively by writing in a clear and structured manner, to evaluate critically investigational or therapeutic strategies and to demonstrate an ability to make considered judgements or recommendations. Do remember to spend time structuring your answer to each question that is being asked and avoid potentially irrelevant areas around that topic that are not pertinent to the examination question being asked.

Paper 2 also lasts 3 hours and contains 125 multiple choice and extended matching (MCQs/EMQs) examining your ability to apply your knowledge over a wide range of subject areas. The questions assess the pathogenesis, investigation and management of haematological disease as well as the use of therapeutic modalities and application of laboratory and clinical practice. 50 questions are "best from 5" format. 75 questions are "extended matching questions (EMQs)" format. No marks are now deducted for an incorrect answer (unlike in my day when the format was based upon the idea that as a clinician we should not be guessing!). Most questions are structured around clinical or laboratory vignettes and are designed to assess your judgement and your ability to apply your knowledge rather than simple recall or recognition of facts. The paper is roughly split so that each of the 4 subject areas is represented in 25% of this examination. A small number of questions may also evaluate your knowledge of management topics, research methodology, ethics or statistics and laboratory management areas such as health and safety, quality assurance and clinical governance. The pass mark for paper 2 is determined by an Angoff procedure, which is a validated method of standard setting by determining minimal acceptable competence and that is approved by the GMC and Academy of Medical Royal Colleges. Under the Angoff method, a panel of subject matter experts (SME) of practicing haematology consultants, provide a rating for each exam question. These SMEs provide a score based on their opinion of the proportion of minimally competent candidates that would score correctly on that item. The judges discuss differences in ratings for the same item and have the opportunity to discuss and modify their ratings. Each independent score is averaged to create an Angoff score for a single question. All of the Angoff scores for each question are combined to create the total score for the examination. So, in essence, this shows not to worry too much about the really hard questions — this will all be ironed out in the methodology used to assess the pass mark for that year's paper.

Now that the examination has been explained, we can get on with passing it. We all have our ways of learning and our own favourite topics and sub-specialization areas, but first you need to know the basics to help get through the examination. Dr Joel McCay has put together the first published book specifically designed to help you pass part 1 and covers all aspects of the haematology curriculum. This wonderful book is a necessity for candidates looking to pass the exam and will be a great addition to your other methods of learning to get you through part 1. Good luck!

Professor John G Gribben MD DSc FRCP FRCPath, FHEA, FMedSci
Hamilton Fairley Chair of Medical Oncology, Barts Cancer Institute, Queen Mary University of London
Honorary Consultant in Haemato-Oncology, St Bartholomew's Hospital, London

Contents

Introduction

Passing the FRCPath Part 1 is a rite of passage for haematology trainees and a source of great anxiety. With over 100 BSH guidelines, 10 Pan-London guidelines and a 3-week transfusion course it is only natural to feel overwhelmed. And this is before we've even talked about coag! My experience of the exam was during the COVID-19 pandemic when courses and teaching were stopped, delayed or moved online making them often harder to attend or not as didactic as face-to-face sessions. Thanks to the advent of online learning these hurdles were slightly easier to overcome but the relentless nature of revision while doing a 1-in-4 on-call rota (if you're lucky) is unsurprisingly too much for many! Though the guidelines for passing the exam are essential, I saw the need for a pocket quick reference guide. There are plenty of excellent revision books or courses out there, but there does not yet exist a quick reference guide with "what to revise as the minimum" for the exam. I would find myself finishing work and getting the tube home, slowly losing concentration as my finger began to cramp from scrolling through the 34-page guideline on rare lymphoid malignancies or platelet function assays on my phone... This was inefficient revision. "A good 30 minutes of revision is better than a poor 4 hours" is something I believe strongly. I have written this guide to encapsulate that mantra.

I envisage this book being used to structure your thoughts when approaching an essay on a topic as well as a quick reminder of certain elements of a topic for the multiple-choice paper. This should not replace reading the guidelines on each! This is an aide-mémoire to the learning you have already gained from your years on the ward and the revision you have already put in. This book will cover the large topics and break them down into need-to-know detail to help you in planning and writing an essay question. There will be sections which I have not covered such as the rarer bleeding disorders or leukaemias. For these, I would advise self-study or attending a course which will cover them.

Each page encompasses the points for writing a good haematology essay to broadly cover a subject. The most salient advice I can pass on came to me from a fellow registrar who had just passed her exam:

"No one cares that you can manage the chronic skin graft versus host disease of a Cy/TBI MUD allograft for relapsed T-ALL with ECP following failed high dose steroids... They want to know you have a broad knowledge on lots of subjects."

List of Abbreviations

-ve: Negative
+ve: Positive
AA: Aplastic anaemia
ABI1: Anti-beta-2 glycoprotein-1 antibody
ACD: Acid, Citrate and Dextrose
ACF: Antecubital fossa
ACL: Anti-cardiolipin antibody
ACR: Albumin creatinine ratio
ACS: Acute chest syndrome
ADAMTS13: A disintegrin and metalloproteinase with thrombospondin type 1 motif, member 13
AHA: Acquired haemophilia A
AHG: Anti-human globulin
AIHA: Autoimmune haemolytic anaemia
AITL: Angioimmunoblastic T-cell lymphoma
ALL: Acute lymphoblastic leukaemia
Allo: Allograft transplant
AML: Acute myeloid leukaemia
Anti-HCV: Anti-Hepatitis C antibody
AP: Accelerated phase
APCC: Activated prothrombin complex concentrate
APML: Acute promyelocytic leukaemia
APS: Antiphospholipid syndrome
APTT: Activated partial thromboplastin time
AT: Anti-Thrombin
ATG: Anti-Thymocyte globulin
ATLL: Adult T-cell leukaemia/lymphoma
Auto: Autograft transplant
AVN: Avascular necrosis
AZT: Zidovudine
B2M: Beta 2 microglobulin
BAT: Bleeding assessment tool
BBB: Blood brain barrier
BBV: Blood borne viruses
BJP: Bence Jones protein
BM: Bone marrow
BMAT: Bone marrow aspirate and trephine
BMFS: Bone marrow failure syndrome
BMT: Bone marrow transplant
BP: Blast phase
BSS: Bernard-Soulier syndrome

BTKi: Bruton's Tyrosine Kinase inhibitor
C1,2,3,4: Consolidation 1,2,3,4
CA: Cold agglutinins
CCF: Chronic congestive heart failure
CCUS: Clonal cytopaenia of undetermined significance
cFDNA: Cell free DNA
CHAD: Cold haemagglutinin disease
CHIP: Clonal haematopoiesis of indeterminate significance
cHL: Classical Hodgkin lymphoma
CHS: Chédiak–Higashi syndrome
CI: Chemo-immunotherapy
CKD: Chronic kidney disease
CLL: Chronic lymphocytic leukaemia
CML: Chronic myeloid leukaemia
CMML: Chronic myelomonocytic leukaemia
CMR: Complete metabolic response
CMUS: Clonal monocytosis of undetermined significance
CMV: Cytomegalovirus
CNS: Central nervous system
CNS-IPI: Central nervous system international prognostic index
COCP: Combine oral contraceptive pill
CP: Chronic phase
CPD: Citrate, Phosphate and Dextrose
CPSS: CMML specific prognostic scoring criteria
CR: Complete response
CR1: Complete remission 1
CR2: Complete remission 2
CrCl: Creatinine clearance calculated by Cockroft-Gault
Cryo: Cryoprecipitate
CSA: Ciclosporin
CSF: Cerebrospinal fluid
CVS: Chorionic villous sampling
DaggT: Direct agglutination test
DAT: Direct antiglobulin test
DC: Dyskeratosis congenita
DIC: Disseminated intravascular coagulopathy
DIPSS: Dynamic international prognostic scoring system
DLBCL: Diffuse large B-cell lymphoma
DOACS: Direct oral anticoagulants
DRVVT: Dilute Russell viper venom test
EATL: Enteropathy associated T-cell lymphoma

EBV: Epstein Barr virus
ECHO: Echocardiogram
ECP: Extracorporeal phosphorylation
ECV: External cephalic version
EORTC: European organisation for research and treatment of cancer
EOTPET: End of treatment PET scan
EPO: Erythropoietin
ESA: Erythropoiesis stimulating agents
ET: Essential thrombocytosis
FA: Fanconi's anaemia
FAB: French and British
FFP: Fresh frozen plasma
FGN: Fibrinogen
FHX: Family history
FID: Functional Iron deficiency
FL: Follicular lymphoma
FLAER: Fluorescein-labelled proaerolysin
FLIPI/FLIPI2: Follicular lymphoma international prognostic index/2
FMH: Fetal maternal haemorrhage
FNHTR: Febrile non-haemolytic transfusion reaction
FOQ: Family of origin questionnaire
FVIII: Factor VIII
GAPC: Gastric anti-parietal antibody
GHSG: German Hodgkin study group
GI: Gastrointestinal
GPI: Glycosylphosphatidylinositol
GPS: Grey platelet syndrome
GU: Genitourinary
Haplo: Haplograft stem cell transplant
HAS: Human albumin solution
HbH: Haemoglobin H
HBsAg: Hepatitis B surface antigen
HBV: Hepatitis B virus
HCC: Hepatocellular carcinoma
HCL/HCL-V: Hairy cell leukaemia/Hairy cell leukaemia variant
HCV: Hepatitis C virus
HDFN: Haemolytic disease of the fetus and newborn
HDM: High dose melphalan
HELLP: Haemolysis, elevated liver enzymes and low platelets
HEV: Hepatitis E virus
HI: Head injury

HIT: Heparin induced thrombocytopaenia
HIV: Human immunodeficiency virus
HLH: Hemophagocytic lymphohistiocytosis
HMW: High molecular weight
HPA: Human platelet antibodies
HPF: High power field
HPLC: High performance liquid chromatography
HPS: Hermansky-Pudlak syndrome
HRC: Hypochromic red cells
HRT: Hormone replacement therapy
HS: Hereditary spherocytosis
HSC: Haematopoietic stem cell
HSCT: Haematopoietic stem cell transplant
HTC: Holotranscobalamin
HTLV1: Human T-lymphotropic virus-1
HTN: Hypertension
HU: Hydroxycarbamide
HUS: Haemolytic uraemic syndrome
IBD: Inflammatory bowel disease
ICB: Intracranial bleed
ICP: Intracranial pressure
ICUS: Idiopathic cytopaenia of undetermined significance
IFAB: Intrinsic factor antibodies
IFN: Interferon alpha
IFRT: Involved field radiotherapy
Ig: Immunoglobulin
IHC: Immunohistochemistry
INR: International normalised ratio
IPD: Inherited platelet disorders
IPI: International prognostic index
IPSS: International prognostic scoring system
IPSS-R: International prognostic scoring system revised
ISI: International sensitivity index
ISSWM: International prognostic scoring system for Waldenström's Macroglobulinaemia
IT: Intrathecal
ITD: Internal tandem duplication
ITI: Immune tolerance induction
IUGR: Intrauterine growth restriction
IUT: Intrauterine transfusion
IV: Intravenous
IVC: inferior vena cava

IVIG: Intravenous immunoglobulin G
IWMG: International working myeloma group
JMML: Juvenile myelomonocytic leukaemia
LA: Lupus anticoagulant
LFTs: Liver function tests
LGL: Large granular lymphocyte
LGLL: Large granulocytic lymphocytic leukaemia
LIMS: Laboratory information management system
LISS: Low ionic strength saline
LMWH: Low molecular weight heparin
LN: Lymph nodes
LP: Lumbar puncture
LTA: Light transmission aggregometry
MAHA: Microangiopathic haemolytic anaemia
MALT: Mucosal associated lymphoid tissue
MBL: Monoclonal B-cell lymphocytosis
MCA: Middle cerebral artery
MDS/MPN-T-*SF3B1*: MDS/MPN with thrombocytosis and *SF3B1* mutation
MDS/MPN-RS-T, NOS: MDS/MPN with ring sideroblasts, thrombocytosis not otherwise specified
MFU: Mycosis Fungoides
MGRS: Monoclonal gammopathy of renal significance
MHA: May-Hegglin anomaly
MIPI: Mantle cell international prognostic index
MiRA: Minor route abnormalities
MM: Multiple myeloma
MMA: Methylmalonic acid
MMF: Mycophenolate mofetil
MOA: Mechanism of action
MPN: Myeloproliferative neoplasm
MPV: Mean platelet volume
MRA: Major route abnormalities
MRD: Minimal residual disease
MSK: Musculoskeletal
MTX: Methotrexate
MUD: Matched unrelated donor
NAT: Nucleic acid testing
NGS: Next generation sequencing
NHL: Non-Hodgkin lymphoma
NHSBT: National Health Service blood and transplant
NLPHL: Nodular lymphocytic predominant Hodgkin Lymphoma

NOS: Not otherwise specified
NRBC: Nucleated red blood cells
NT-proBNP: N-Terminal prohormone of brain natriuretic peptide
NYHA: New York Heart Association
OGD: Gastroscopy
ORR: Overall response rate
OS: Overall survival
PA: Purine analogue
PAD: Pre-deposit autologous donation
PAS: Platelet additive solution
PB: Peripheral blood
PCC: Prothrombin complex concentrate
PCH: Paroxysmal cold haemoglobinuria
PCNSL: Primary CNS lymphoma
PCR: Protein creatinine ratio
Peg-IFN: Pegylated interferon
PEP: Post-exposure prophylaxis
PF4: Platelet factor 4
PFA-100/200: Platelet function assay 100/200
PFS: Progression free survival
Ph: Philadelphia chromosome
PI: Proteasome inhibitor
PID: Pelvic inflammatory disease
PLEX: Plasma exchange
PMBCL: Primary mediastinal B-cell lymphoma
PNH: Paroxysmal nocturnal haemoglobinuria
POEMS: Polyneuropathy, Organomegaly, Endocrinopathy, Monoclonal gammopathy and Skin
PP: Paraprotein
PPP: Platelet poor plasma
PPH: Postpartum haemorrhage
PPI: Proton pump inhibitor
PR: Partial response
PrEP: Pre-exposure prophylaxis
PRP: Platelet rich plasma
PS: Performance status
PT: Prothrombin time
PTR: Prothrombin ratio
PTP: Post-transfusion purpura
PUVA: Psoralen ultraviolet light A
QOL: Quality of life

R/R: Relapsed/Refractory
RA: Rheumatoid arthritis
RD: Refractory disease
Rh: Rhesus
RIC: Reduced intensity conditioning
RIPA: Ristocetin induced platelet agglutination
RT: Richter's transformation
Rt-PCR: Real time-Polymerase chain reaction
RTX: Radiotherapy
S/D FFP: Solvent detergent fresh frozen plasma
SACT: Systemic anticancer treatment
SAG-M: Saline, Adenine, Glucose and Mannitol
SAP: Serum amyloid protein
SBDS: Schwachman-Bodian-Diamond syndrome
SCA: Sickle cell anaemia
sCR: Stringent complete response
SD: Stable disease
SDS: Schwachman-Diamond syndrome
SDS: Solvent detergent solution
SE: Southeast
SFLC: Serum free light chains
SHOT: Serious hazards of transfusion
SLE: Systemic lupus erythematosus
SLL: Small lymphocytic leukaemia
SM-AHN: Systemic mastocytosis with associated haematological neoplasm
SMZL: Splenic marginal zone lymphoma
SOB: Shortness of breath
SVC: Superior vena cava
SVCO: Superior vena cava obstruction
SYK: Spleen tyrosine kinase
TA-GvHD: Transfusion associated graft versus host disease
TACO: Transfusion associated circulatory overload
TCR: T-cell receptor
TF: Tissue factor
TIPSS: Transjugular intrahepatic portosystemic shunt
TKD: Tyrosine kinase domain
TLS: Tumour lysis syndrome
TPO-RA: Thrombopoietin receptor agonist
TRALI: Transfusion related acute lung injury
TRV: Tricuspid regurgitation velocity
TSAT: Transferrin saturation

TT: Thrombin time
TTP: Thrombotic thrombocytopenic purpura
Tx: Treatment
TXA: Tranexamic acid
TYA: Teenagers, youths and adolescents
UC: Ulcerative colitis
UF: Ultrafiltration
UFH: Unfractionated heparin
UGI: Upper gastrointestinal
ULN: Upper limit of normal
USS: Ultrasound scan
VAF: Variant allele frequency
vCJD: Variant Creutzfeldt-Jakob disease
VITT: Vaccine-induced immune thrombocytopaenia and thrombosis
VOD: Vaso-occlusive disease
VTE: Venous thromboembolism
VWD: Von Willebrand disease
VWF: Von Willebrand factor
WB: Whole blood
WBIT: Wrong blood in tube
WCC: White cell count
WHO: World Health Organisation
WM: Waldenström's macroglobulinaemia
ZPP: Zinc Protoporphyrin

How to Use This Book

A few bullet points on how to use the book and themes throughout which may not be ubiquitous with all trainees either in the UK or from overseas.

- Figures such as OS and PFS have been rounded or averaged from multiple guidelines to give a flavour of the average expected outcomes. I tried to make it as if you were speaking to a patient in clinic. You wouldn't (you might but it's a bit odd) say "your chances of 5-year OS are 33.7%"; you'd say something like "30–40%".
- I've used a lot of abbreviations in the book which are above. Some are very common, some less so.
- The layout for the majority of the subjects is designed to be essay format. This is more common in the haematological malignancy section and less so in the lab aspects of the other domains. I have made it an essay plan layout where possible, but some subjects are easier than others to lay out in this way.
- Even though the purpose of the book is to be a pocket guide for revising for the exam, I've tried to make it relevant and useful for new ST3 registrars being on the ward. I have not included every ounce of detail on the various subtypes and trial treatments available in all disorders. For new treatments and very specific detail, use: BSH guidelines, good practice papers and attended MDT meetings.
- There will be some crossover between sections within the book, but this should be minimal.
- Chemotherapy regimens, such as R-CHOP, are assumed to be known. If not known, look them up. Common medical terms, such as ECHO or SOB, are assumed knowledge. Any abbreviated drugs, such as HU for hydroxycarbamide will be in the abbreviations section. Molecular abbreviations, such as *NOTCH3*, will be assumed and the exact scientific name should be looked up externally.
- BSH guidelines or pan-London guidelines are generally the ones I've referenced but there is also a lot of WHO and international consensus committee guidance used in the Haematological Oncology section.
- Genes are in italics and the protein they encode are not i.e., "*ALK* mutated gene in ALCL causing overexpression of the ALK protein".
- Finally, it might feel that there is a huge amount of detail to know for the exam. Anyone who says they know it all is lying or is a genius; but more likely lying. I've worked with world-renowned consultants who still refresh their memory and look up the guidelines for the nitty gritty, rare scenarios or new protocols. Please do not worry. There are parts in the book where I have said "high risk features" and have not listed them. It would be worth knowing 1 or 2 but my goal was not to create an all-knowing guide to every single detail in every single guideline. For those who want to know more I have included further reading at the end of each subject and references at the end of the book with some interesting, good practice papers or large studies, but these are not essential.

Exam Tips

This handbook should not replace the essential British Society of Haematology guidelines (I know I am banging on about this, but it really should not!); I would recommend reading all of them at least once. Some are wordier than others and some hold more relevance to clinical practice than what may be asked in an exam paper. They can seem quite daunting at first but planning your revision schedule is key. My top tips for a successful revision period and passing the exam are as follows.

1. Plan your revision and allow good time

It may sound daft but plan your revision timeline! You'll start with the best intentions of working every day and weekend but that will not happen. On calls, long days, nights, leave and children will all impact on your ability to revise. You want to allow a good amount of time to cover everything once but also not too long where you will run out of steam. As a rule of thumb, I would say allow 4 months of time from the start of revision to the exam date. I would also allow 2–3 weeks at the end to purely practise exam technique and get "match fit" for the big day.

2. Accept your revision will vary based on your rota

This is not an undergraduate exam where you have ample daytime hours to prep. You must accept that your work will unfortunately come first and often days you had planned to do a few hours revision where you are covering the lab may get lost to clinical commitments. Equally, planning to work on the commute home or in the evening is not always feasible or beneficial after a busy day. Allowing yourself to be flexible day-to-day and not being hard on yourself if you don't get as much done as you'd planned is crucial. Take it a step at a time and try not to overthink the bigger picture.

3. Start with something you enjoy

A subject you enjoy and are familiar with is a good starting point rather than diving into something complex and "heavy". It's also a good way to familiarise yourself with the guideline structure and length. Some of them are very lab-based and I would say it's best to save these until the peak of your revision when you are more efficient at reading and processing these lengthy guidelines. Equally, unless you are really interested in something I would say to focus on the bullet pointed bold summaries of the guidelines rather than the intricate literature reviews or the multiple trials behind these guidelines. It is good to have 1 trial you can quote but this is the cherry on top when writing an essay and is much less important than having a broad knowledge on a particular subject.

4. Request study leave early and speak to your educational supervisor

This is important and your rota co-ordinator will thank you for letting them know early! As well as leave for the exam and courses, you are *entitled* to some private study days as well. Though you are entitled to these study days, clinical duties may take precedence; advanced notice to your rota co-ordinator will ensure you get the time you need. It's also wise to let your head of department or educational supervisor know in advance for pastoral support. Finally, if you're lucky, you may be able to request certain job roles with less clinical pressure to allow for extra revision time or a role where you feel you could do with some support in your development and revision. Speaking to the rota team and heads of department early is advised should you wish to do this.

5. Form a revision group

Though it may feel daunting, a revision group is a good way to find your blind spots or areas which you need to work on. As well as aiding your learning it provides a good way of letting off steam with your colleagues and supporting each other. These groups are particularly useful towards the end of your revision and as a group you can divide a paper up, answer a section and then come back together to discuss each part. I found this an effective way of covering the vast number of past papers that are out there. Relying on other registrars who have sat the exam for tips and tricks is also incredibly useful as they have been through what you are going through now.

6. Mix up your revision style

A key reason I thought this book would be useful was to use it as a pocket guide, a bit like some of the other specialty revision books that are out there, to mix up revision styles and keep it varied. Question banks are great for when you have 15–30 minutes and feel like you want to test your knowledge. Podcasts are great for doing revision while making dinner or exercising and there are loads of great ones out there. BSH and ASH also do lecture series they release as a podcast on updates in haematology. Bottom line: Mix it up.

7. Plan writing essays

This is a massive issue that lots of people tend to have problems with when taking the exam. Given that most of our undergraduate and postgraduate exams have been multiple choice it is not surprising that constructing an essay in a short period of time can be challenging for us. Even those who are used to writing essays can find compiling their thoughts and knowledge on a topic difficult in 45 minutes. Practice is key here.

Essay planning is essential and can be applied to all the topics, but I would advise watching some YouTube tutorials on this as well as tricks to get your points across. One of the pitfalls I fell into when revising was the following:

"Describe the current treatment indications, rationale and regimes for a patient referred to you with a confirmed diagnosis of CLL (10 marks)"
- Proceeds to write any interesting point about CLL as well as rambling about CLL score, experimental treatments, BTK inhibitor resistance and Richter's transformation.
- Realises I've spent 20 minutes bigging up my understanding of CLL and its intricacies and not mentioned anything about treatment.
- Bullet points all known CLL treatments as acronyms without explaining the indications for and against treatment as well as specifics.
- Runs out of time.

This is quite a common problem and essay planning can get around this. Get to the crux of what the question is asking you and even write this part first! Then fill around it with the fluffy detail which makes a good essay.

8. Ample breaks

Again, this sounds obvious, but people don't take a break and think that more hours revising equates to more knowledge. A "good" hour is better than 4 "OK" hours re-reading the same paragraph from the follicular lymphoma guideline on the different progression-free survival rates in maintenance therapy. If you aren't absorbing something just leave it and come back to it. I covered Bethesda assays roughly 9 times repeatedly without any success, wasting about 6 hours of my life. It stressed me out beyond belief. Some weeks later an ST7 I was working with explained it to me in 15 minutes and it clicked. If you persevere with something which is still causing you stress and you can't grasp, take this advice. Stop. Reassess. Reach out for help. It's important to allow yourself downtime as well. Still go out and socialise with friends and family, have days off where you do nothing and find positive ways to relax. You'll come back stronger and recharged the next day. It's a marathon not a sprint.

9. Courses

There are a few courses out there and though they are quite intense and normally on a weekend, I do think they're useful. I would recommend doing them about 2–4 weeks before your exam (if that's possible) to highlight your blind spots. They also cover loads of areas that aren't in the guidelines that are quite niche. But don't worry, these are more useful for the multiple-choice paper rather than the essays. It's very unlikely they'll ask you to write an essay on blastic plasmacytoid dendritic neoplasms, but they might ask you the characteristic flow panel (CD123, CD4, CD56 "123456"). It's not worth your time revising all of these but the courses offer good coverage of the more common of the uncommon ones you may encounter.

10. Previous exam papers

This is a must and you're a fool if you don't do your research. It may sound obvious, but it is very unlikely that the paper from the last sitting featuring a TTP question will have another one in the upcoming exam. Equally, if CML has not appeared in an essay in 7–8 years there may be a good chance it will appear in your exam. This doesn't mean you should disregard everything else but work smart when it comes to revising your weak areas, especially if they have not appeared in the exam for some time. Equally, if you are strong on an area which appeared in the last exam it might not be worth investing much more revision time in said topic.

Red Cell Haematology

Red cell haematology is commonly overlooked for the exam with many people putting more effort into the coagulation and haematological oncology sections. For that reason, people often can come unstuck when writing a red cell essay and struggle to formulate a well-rounded answer. I have therefore started with red cell to help avoid this common pitfall. The structure for each section will generally follow a pattern similar to how you would write an essay. Most sections will start with an introduction and epidemiology section which I think is always a good nerve settler and springboard for writing an essay on any topic. Some topics will have sections which repeat and for those please refer to the sections above if not mentioned, such as the case in the haemoglobinopathies. The aim of the structure is for revising topics quickly in a more condensed format compared to the guidelines, but also to structure your thought process on how to approach an essay question. For example, you may have a question "Describe how you would risk-stratify patients with sickle cell anaemia in clinic". For this, I do not advise just regurgitating the whole HbSS section from the book but to structure it as follows:

1. Introduction.
2. Epidemiology.
3. Brief pathophysiology.
4. Common symptoms of sickle cell anaemia.
5. Acute presentations which classify patients as high risk/poorly managed disease.
6. Chronic presentations which classify patients as high risk/poorly managed disease.
7. Side effects of treatment which make patients high risk.
8. Other comments and conclusions.

At no point in the structure of this essay have I ever really touched on the management or in-depth genetic origins of sickle cell anaemia. Though interesting and a need-to-know for the exam it is not required in this question.

The point I am trying to make: READ THE QUESTION CAREFULLY AND ANSWER IT PRECISELY!

Haemoglobinopathies and Thalassaemia

Sickle Cell Disease (HbSS)

Introduction: Sickle cell disease is a haemoglobinopathy due to an amino acid substitute leading to abnormal haemoglobin formation. There are various mutations which can occur leading to a variety of new haemoglobin molecule formations which classifies each disease differently. Haemoglobin SS disease is due to homozygous mutation in the beta globin gene causing an abnormal haem molecule.

Epidemiology: Commonly affects Africans as well as other ethnicities including Central and South Americans of partly African ethnicity, Greek, Turkish, Arabic and Indian populations. Median overall survival age is 65. Multiple chronic health problems associated such as stroke, lung, renal or bone disease as well as increased mortality rates due to acute complications like acute chest syndrome, aplastic anaemia, infection or hepatic and splenic sickle disease. Affects 1:2,500 births.

Signs/symptoms: Anaemia, painful crisis, splenomegaly, failure to thrive, strokes or thrombosis, infections and avascular necrosis.

FBC: Commonly microcytic anaemia with raised RDW, reticulocytosis and typically abnormal red cell indices. Anaemia often 60–90 g/L.

Blood film: Sickle cells, target cells, fragments, crenated cells, Howell-Jolly bodies, Heinz bodies and anisopoikilocytosis.

Diagnosis: Antenatal screening done on all UK-born babies who fall into high-risk category on the FOQ.

Consider pre-surgery screening in high-risk populations due to risk of anaesthesia causing acute crisis. Done in IVF treatment routinely.

Postnatal screening on all babies arriving in the UK under the age of 1. Consider in patients with unexplained anaemia from high-prevalence area. Part of the new-born heel prick test performed around 5 days old.

"The presence of abnormal haemoglobin by diagnostic test and confirmed by another method such as sickle solubility test".

2 +ve tests to confirm diagnosis as an abnormal haemoglobin could be trait, not disease. Presence of HbS and no or minimal HbA seen on HPLC or haemoglobin electrophoresis in disease. Often HbS > 80%.

Pathophysiology: HbA is the primary Hb by 3–6 months in healthy babies. In sickle cell disease the abnormal Hb molecule will be present instead of HbA, hence symptoms may occur at this point. HbF remains in the circulation, though diminishing, until 6 months where it makes up 2–3% of total Hb and therefore symptoms may not occur until then. Mutation of the beta globin gene leads to formation of haemoglobin S, in SS this is homozygous. This leads to deformed sickled red cells which causes chronic haemolytic anaemia and vaso-occlusion which causes symptoms and organ damage.

Molecular: Mutated beta globin gene. Single base mutation leads to valine rather than glutamic acid in position 6 of 147 amino acid chain.

Tx at diagnosis? Yes, all will receive supportive care with penicillin V, folic acid, COVID-19 vaccinations, seasonal flu vaccination, pneumovax every 5 years and meningitis B, C and ACWY. ECHO for cardiac disease every 3 years. Slit lamp exam and urinary PCR for retinal and renal disease respectively. Regular follow up in clinic to manage complications, prevent hospital admissions and emergency scenarios.

Other important work up:

At diagnosis: Family history, siblings who are affected, red cell phenotyping, screen for BBV namely Hep B, C and HIV, G6PD, HbS%.

At regular clinic appointments: Ferritin to consider iron chelation. If > 1000 ug/ml to arrange a Ferriscan and T2 cardiac MRI and offer iron chelation based on results (if liver iron > 7 mg/gDW). Regular urine PCR ensuring < 50 mg/mmol. ECHO every 3 years looking at TRV and ensuring < 2.5 m/s. Lung function tests for pulmonary hypertension if symptoms. HbS% regularly. Vitamin D. TCD in children to look at MCA pressures yearly.

Disease modifying therapy:

HU: Offered from 9–42 months regardless of disease severity, in all with 3 or more acute complications within a year, in all who have severe phenotype or all who have had ACS. Can use as primary stroke prevention in children who have had 1 year of regular transfusions without imaging associated cerebral vasculopathy.

If someone has had a stroke, then a red cell exchange programme should be used.

HU works by increasing HbF production, decreased expression of adhesion molecules and increases vasodilation by nitric oxide donation.

Side effects of HU: Fertility preservation in young adults, leg ulcers, teratogenicity, cytopaenias and requires regular monitoring.

Regular red cell exchange programme: Performed when someone has had a stroke or intolerant of HU as secondary stroke prophylaxis. Commonly red cell exchange done once a month as a rule of thumb, though does vary. Top up transfusion also used in these patients.

Specific scenarios:

ACS: Fever, respiratory symptoms and CXR changes. Sats < 94% or drop from baseline of 3%. PaO2 < 8 kPa then exchange.

Can buy some time with top up transfusions and NIV but if Hb > 90 g/L, needs urgent exchange. High mortality and emergency scenario. Risk of fat embolism also and ACS can be preceded by infection or painful crisis.

Treatment: IVF, incentive spirometry, analgesia, red cell exchange, prophylactic anticoagulation, ITU support and broad-spectrum antibiotics including a macrolide.

Sequestration: Pooling of blood in spleen or liver.

Splenic sequestration more common in children and presents with splenomegaly, pallor, shock.

Treatment: Broad-spectrum IV antibiotics and RBC transfusion.

Intrahepatic cholestasis: Abdominal pain and raised liver function tests.

Treatment: Red cell exchange transfusion.

Painful crisis: Severe bone and joint pain. Can occur with or without a trigger.

Well recognised triggers include cold weather, infection, hypoxia, dehydration, pregnancy and menstruation.

Treatment: IVF, antibiotics, analgesia within 30 minutes of presentation, oxygen and warming.

Aplastic: Pancytopaenia, fever, reticulocytopaenia and splenomegaly, commonly due to Parvovirus B19.

Treatment: Transfuse, supportive care and screen other family members with sickle cell disease for Parvovirus.

Pregnancy: Counselling pre-conception and partner testing.

Complications include VTE, UTI, spontaneous abortion, pre-eclampsia, preterm delivery and IUGR.

Start: Vit D, Folic acid and penicillin V. Ensure vaccinations are up to date including seasonal flu and COVID-19.

Ensure up to date with screening tests i.e., recent echo, ophthalmology review. Low dose aspirin from 12–36 weeks' gestation. Thromboprophylaxis from 28 weeks' gestation and 6 weeks postpartum. If additional risk factors, start earlier in pregnancy. Monitor regularly in a specialist combined obstetric haematology clinic. Serial growth scans with dopplers every 4 weeks from 24 weeks.

Stop: HU, ACE inhibitor and iron chelation, ideally 3 months prior to conception.

Increased risk of sickle specific complications, such as painful crises, and ACS.

Consider: Transfusion with ABO, RH, Kell matched CMV -ve blood in select cases.

Birth: In hospital, any mode of delivery, keep warm, regional analgesia and opioids ok to use but there is always a risk/reward benefit to consider.

Post: LMWH for 6 weeks and monitor as high risk for painful crisis.

Indications for urgent red cell exchange: Acute neurological events, ACS, multi-organ failure, severe sepsis, systemic fat embolism, progressive hepatopathy, resistant priapism, surgery, girdle syndrome, emergency surgery or endoscopic intervention.

Indications for an elective red cell exchange programme: Primary stroke prevention in patients transitioning from paediatrics, secondary stroke prevention, pregnancy if maternal sickle related complications, leg ulcers refractory to other measures.

Goals of exchange: 8–10 units of RBC aiming to drop HbS% < 30 (20 in stroke or if critically unwell) and haemoglobin 100–110 g/L with target HCT 0.32–0.34.

Other treatments:

<u>HSCT</u>: Young with severe disease and appropriate unaffected matched sibling donor. REDRESS trial is a randomised trial looking at haploidentical transplants in sickle cell disease.

<u>Volexetor</u>: HbS polymerization inhibitor preventing adhesion and sickling by increasing HbS affinity for oxygen. Not NICE approved.

<u>CRISPR-Cas9</u>: Targets beta globin gene abnormality via viral vector and knocks out gene. Now FDA approved.

Supportive care:

<u>Infections</u>: Penicillin V and vaccination for hyposplenism.

<u>Bone disease</u>: Vitamin D and regular monitoring for AVN. Ortho review if AVN.

<u>Stroke</u>: Aspirin if history of stroke and be aware of increased risk of vascular dementia.

<u>Liver disease</u>: Regular medication review and monitoring for cholestasis or iron overload.

<u>Iron chelation</u>: Regular monitoring and Ferriscan if raised TSAT. Consider chelation if on long-term regular exchange programme.

Monitor joints for signs of iron deposition as very disabling if occurs.

<u>Analgesia</u>: At home analgesia in case of mild painful crisis.

<u>Clinical psychologist</u>: Chronic disease, which is very disabling, important to involve early and important in those with opiate dependence.

<u>Antibody formation</u>: Regular antibody screening. ABO, Rh and Kell matched blood.

<u>Priapism</u>: Vasodilators and urology discussion.

Other considerations: Haemoglobinopathy and antibody cards, can tolerate low haemoglobin so empower patient to know their steady state Hb and other numbers, warm clothing and avoiding the cold if possible, contraception in women of childbearing age or hormone therapy to manage menstruation and prevent exacerbation of crisis.

Guidelines:

https://onlinelibrary.wiley.com/doi/full/10.1111/j.1365-2141.2009.08054.x

https://onlinelibrary.wiley.com/doi/full/10.1111/bjh.15235

https://onlinelibrary.wiley.com/doi/full/10.1111/bjh.13348

https://onlinelibrary.wiley.com/doi/full/10.1111/bjh.17671

Sickle Cell Disease (HbSC)

Many sections are the same as above or similar. If the section is not mentioned below, please refer to HbSS section above.

Introduction: HbSC sickle cell disease is characterised by the presence of the 2 abnormal haemoglobin molecules HbS and HbC.

Epidemiology: Considered less aggressive in phenotype with less complications and therefore better median OS.

Common in west African populations as well as Mediterranean and Caribbean.

Signs/symptoms: Generally, symptoms and crisis are less frequent and milder than SS disease. Commonly retinopathy, renal and bone disease are the major problems. Often splenomegaly more pronounced compared to HbSS.

FBC: Anaemia not as severe, often between 80–120 g/L. MCV and MCH lower than HbSS.

Blood film: SC poikilocytes and SC crystal seen, which are irregular shaped haemoglobin crystals within red cells. SC poikilocytes resemble sickled cells with "branches" or "protrusions" from the membrane. As above feature of HbSS disease also seen such as haemolysis and hyposplenism.

Diagnosis: Presence of HbS and C on HPLC and confirmed by second screening test. Often 40–45% each with minimal or no HbA.

Molecular: Compound mutation in the beta globin gene leading to HbS formation as mentioned above combined with a separate point mutation leading to amino acid substation of lysine for glutamic acid in the other globin chain.

Tx at diagnosis? Yes, same considerations as above though all treatment and trials generally based on HbSS disease. In clinical practice apply the same treatment goals to HbSC disease. In red cell exchange and steady state haemoglobin the Hb targets will be different as baseline generally higher.

Other important work up: As above.

First line tx options: As above.

Emergency scenarios: As above.

Supportive care: As above.

Other considerations: Same follow up and MDT as other haemoglobinopathies and even though "milder" phenotype, some patients can still have troubling symptoms and disabling chronic disease.

Guidelines: As above.

Sickle Cell Trait (HbAS)

Introduction: Caused by inheriting 1 abnormal globin gene associated with sickle cell disease and 1 normal haemoglobin gene.

Epidemiology: More common than disease. Around 300 million people worldwide have sickle cell trait. No effect on life expectancy.

Signs/symptoms: Asymptomatic, picked up due to family screening, prenatal testing or through other health screening. May get symptoms at high altitude, or low oxygen states. Be aware during ITU admissions or anaesthesia but very rare.

FBC/Blood film: Often normal though occasionally mild reduction in MCV.

Diagnosis: HbS present but < 50% and HbA > 50% with no anaemia. Sickle cell solubility test will likely be +ve if HbS % > 15–20.

Molecular: Heterozygous mutation in gene associated with SCD with the other gene producing a normal Hb molecule.

Tx at diagnosis? No, rare established complications include renal medullary carcinoma, splenic infarcts at high altitude but generally none.

Other considerations: Important for family planning.

Alpha Thalassaemia

Introduction: Reduced or absent production of haemoglobin alpha globin chains due to mutation or deletion which results in an imbalance in beta globin chain production causing haemolysis, anaemia and extramedullary haematopoiesis in HbH disease. Can co-exist with haemoglobinopathies producing a variety of phenotypes.

Epidemiology: Higher prevalence in malaria endemic areas, African, Southeast Asian, Greek, Indian, Mediterranean and Middle Eastern.

Signs/symptoms: HbH have symptomatic anaemia, jaundice, leg ulcers, splenomegaly, infections and failure to thrive in children.

FBC: Low MCV and MCH. In trait only mild reduction and borderline Hb. MCH 25–27 pg, consider carrier state. In HbH disease there is anaemia, MCV < 75 fL and MCH normally < 25 pg with symptoms such as splenomegaly, anaemia and Jaundice. Hb 80–100 g/L in HbH. Normal Hb in trait affecting 1 gene, borderline in trait affecting 2 genes.

Blood film: Target cells, NRBC, reticulocytes and a microcytic, hypochromic picture, red cell inclusions.

Diagnosis: Consider if anaemic with low MCV, MCH and raised RDW and RBC from endemic area or family history or higher risk ethnic group. HPLC shows HbA < 3.5% in trait and < 1.5% in HbH disease and mild increase in HbA$_2$. HbH peak detected on HPLC as a haemoglobin variant. Screening generally done based on FOQ and if family history done at 12–18 weeks via CVS.

Pathophysiology: Excess beta globin chain production leads to ineffective haemo-globin molecule formation which is unstable and precipitates within the red cell. This leads to abnormal red cells causing haemolysis and reduced lifespan and ineffective haematopoiesis. This occurs in HbH and in hydrops fetalis it is so severe that it is not compatible with life. Carrier states have no pathophysiological complications listed above.

Molecular: Generally larger deletions rather than single point mutations affecting genes identified on chromosome 16.

Trait: Either 1 gene on 1 chromosome, 1 gene on each chromosome or 2 genes on 1 chromosome.

HbH disease: 3 alpha genes affected.

Hb Bart's hydrops fetalis: All 4 genes affected.

Tx at diagnosis? Not unless HbH disease. Treatment is usually with transfusion support to suppress endogenous abnormal Hb production if needed. Hugely variable condition. Non-deletional HbH tends to be more severe. No curative options though ongoing trials with agents such as Mitapivat used in PK deficiency.

Other important work up: Exclude other causes of anaemia i.e., iron deficiency or of chronic disease, ECHO, G6PD screening, red cell extended phenotype, DEXA scan as increased risk of osteoporosis in HbH disease.

Supportive care: Often patient need no supportive care if asymptomatic. Those who do require supportive care: Consider folic acid supplements, iron chelation with either subcutaneous or oral agents based on regular ferritin screening, analgesia, bone protection with vitamin D or bisphosphonate. Rh and ABO typed blood, ECHO for regular pulmonary hypertension screening and cardiac follow up if needed, monitoring for endocrinopathies if raised ferritin and iron overload status.

Guidelines:

https://onlinelibrary.wiley.com/doi/full/10.1111/j.1365-2141.2009.08054.x

https://ashpublications.org/blood/article/118/13/3479/29247/How-I-treat-thalassemia

Beta Thalassaemia

Introduction: Reduced or absent production of haemoglobin beta globin chains due to mutation or deletion which results in an imbalance in alpha globin chain production causing haemolysis, anaemia and extramedullary haematopoiesis in beta thalassaemia major. Beta thalassaemia trait is asymptomatic without any of the complications mentioned above. Beta thalassaemia intermedia has a spectrum of symptoms and variable phenotypes. Beta thalassaemia can also co-exist with haemoglobinopathies.

Epidemiology: As above for alpha but more broad spread. Around 100 million people are carriers.

Signs/symptoms: Symptomatic anaemia, jaundice, hepatosplenomegaly, leg ulcers, extramedullary haematopoiesis leading to expanded bone marrow and bone deformities affecting sinuses, long bones and skull, infection, lymphadenopathy. Failure to thrive in children in beta thalassaemia major.

FBC: Chronic microcytic hypochromic anaemia, MCV and MCH reduced, worse in intermedia or major.

<u>Minor</u>: Borderline anaemia, generally Hb > 100 g/l and MCV < 75 fL, MCH 25–27 pg.

<u>Intermedia or major</u>: Both have MCV < 75 fL and MCH < 25 pg with Hb 70–90 g/L and < 70 g/L respectively.

Blood film: Microcytic, hypochromic anaemia with basophilic stippling, red cell inclusions and target cells.

<u>Intermedia or major</u>: As above + reticulocytosis, anisopoikilocytosis and NRBC.

Diagnosis: Anaemic with low MCV, MCH and raised RDW and RBC from endemic area, family history or higher risk ethnic group. HPLC shows predominantly HbF with mild elevation in HbA_2 in major and no HbA. Less pronounced in intermedia. HbA_2 generally > 4% in trait with small amount of HbA. Screening generally done based on FOQ and if family history investigated at 12–18 weeks via CVS.

Pathophysiology: Excess alpha globin chain production leads to ineffective haemoglobin molecule formation which is unstable and precipitates within the red cell. This causes abnormal red cells causing haemolysis and reduced lifespan and ineffective haematopoiesis. Hb variant forms from alpha and gamma globin production characterised by HbF peak on HPLC. Often erythroid hyperplasia on BM biopsy.

Molecular: There are only 2 beta globin genes per cell compared to 4 alpha globin genes. Abnormalities affecting chromosome 11. Generally due to single point mutations resulting in reduced or absent beta globin synthesis. More than 200 identified.

Tx at diagnosis? Not in trait, depends on phenotype of beta thalassaemia intermedia. Generally, intermedia or major treated, monitored and followed up in clinic.

Other important work up: Iron status or other causes of chronic anaemia. Iron deficiency will lead to minor reduction in HbA_2 and can be misleading especially in diagnosis of beta thalassaemia minor.

For intermedia and major: Red cell extended phenotype, NGS to establish mutations, ECHO, G6PD, vitamin D, urine PCR, DEXA scan. If ferritin > 500 ng/ml then T2 cardiac MRI, Ferriscan and screen for endocrinopathies.

Goals of treatment: Intermedia have a variable phenotype some need no transfusions at all, it's a nuanced decision process. Based on severity of anaemia (Hb < 70 g/L), symptoms, evidence of cardiac failure or other significant co-morbidities. May need one-off transfusion if isolated Hb fall and important to rule out other causes for anaemia in those scenarios i.e., iron deficiency. Thalassaemia major need transfusions to survive with the aim of a pre-transfusion Hb of 95–100 g/l to inhibit bone marrow expansion, minimise iron loading and promote normal growth. New guidance from the Thalassaemia International Federation target of > 100 g/L.

Curative treatments:

Allograft: Ideally from matched sibling, MUD if not. Disease free survival > 90% with TRM < 5% and chronic GvHD around 5%.

CRISPR-CAS9: Gene editing using viral vector to introduce genetically modified code into CD34+ HSC which then restores gamma globin synthesis and increases HbF production.

Important side effects of tx: Allo and autoimmunisation, iron overload, transfusion reactions, GvHD from transplant and TRM from infections or conditioning, CRISPR-CAS9 risk include the same as allograft and off-target genome editing.

Supportive care: As above for alpha thalassaemia.

Guidelines:

https://onlinelibrary.wiley.com/doi/full/10.1111/j.1365-2141.2009.08054.x

https://ashpublications.org/blood/article/118/13/3479/29247/How-I-treat-thalassemia

Other Haemoglobinopathies or Thalassaemia Variants

A short summary on some (not all) of the more common or relevant for the exam

HbC Disease

Introduction: Disorder affecting beta globin gene due to glutamic acid substitution with lysine at position 6 commonly affecting West Africans.
Symptoms: Splenomegaly, cholelithiasis, mild anaemia and jaundice. Varying range of symptoms in disease based on severity. None in trait.
Diagnosis: Low MCV and MCH, reticulocytes, target cells and HbC crystals in red cell. HPLC shows HbC peak, HbF and absent HbA in HbC disease but not in trait.
Treatment: Mild chronic haemolytic anaemia in homozygous disease. Support with folic acid. Worse with coexisting haemoglobinopathy.

HbD Disease

Introduction: Disorder affecting beta globin gene due to glutamic acid substitution with lysine at position 121 commonly affecting Indians.
Symptoms: Mild anaemia and jaundice, splenomegaly in disease. None in trait.
Diagnosis: Mild anaemia and target cells. HPLC demonstrates peak in HbD window and low HbA.
Treatment: Often none needed if heterozygous. Homozygous mild phenotype. Clinically significant if inherited with other haemoglobinopathy especially HbS.

HbE Disease

Introduction: Disorder affecting beta globin gene due to glutamic acid substitution with lysine at position 26 commonly affecting Southeast Asians.
Symptoms: Trait: Asymptomatic. Homozygous: Mild haemolytic anaemia. Combined with HbS or beta thalassaemia: Most severe forms with acute and chronic complication in HbE/beta thalassaemia and increased morbidity and mortality.
Diagnosis: Mild anaemia (lower with beta thalassaemia), low MCV and MCH. HPLC peak at HbA_2. Trait: > 3%. Disease: > 10%.
Treatment: Avoid oxidants or precipitants, transfusion if severe symptomatic anaemia.

HPFH

Introduction: Disorder affecting beta or gamma globin chains with increased and imbalanced gamma chain production increasing HbF.

Symptoms: Often asymptomatic even when HbF 100%. Commonly affecting Greek or African populations.

Diagnosis: Very mild anaemia with normal red cell indices. HbF > 20% normally and in homozygous 100%. Important to make diagnosis antenatally as postnatally child may be labelled as HbSS due to high HbF and absence of HbA until 6 months.

Treatment: None needed unless inherited with beta thalassaemia.

Delta Beta Thalassaemia

Introduction: Disorder affecting beta and delta globin chains leading to reduced or absent production.

Symptoms: Considered similar to phenotype of beta thalassaemia minor or intermedia and generally milder than major.

Diagnosis: Microcytic anaemia varying based on hetero or homozygous. HPLC shows elevated HbF and reduced HbA and HbA_2.

Treatment: Transfusion support only really needed if inherited with beta thalassaemia or HbS.

Gamma Delta Beta Thalassaemia

Introduction: Disorder affecting gamma, beta and delta globin chains leading to reduced or absent production. Homozygous mutations lead to stillbirth.

Symptoms: Severe neonatal haemolysis, resolves after HbF production stops at 3 months and less severe phenotype in adults.

Diagnosis: Haemolytic anaemias in neonates. Adults similar to beta thalassaemia trait phenotype. HPLC in adults normal HbF and HbA_2.

Treatment: Transfusion support generally only needed in neonatal period.

HB Lepore

Introduction: Crossover of beta and delta globin genes leading to inefficient globin production which results in trait or disease.

Symptoms: None in trait. In disease the phenotype is broad with some requiring regular transfusion due to severe anaemia.

Diagnosis:

Trait: HbA 80–90%, HbF 1–3%, HbA_2 2–2.5%, Hb Lepore 9–11%.

Disease: HbA 0%, HbF 70–90%, HbA_2 0%, Hb Lepore 8–30%.

Treatment: Transfusion in those with disease who have severe phenotype or when combined with other haemoglobinopathy or thalassaemia.

Hb Constant Spring

Introduction: Disorder due to mutation in the alpha globin gene leading to an elongated alpha globin chain and formation of the unstable haemoglobin HbCS.

Symptoms: Homozygous have mild anaemia like thalassaemia intermedia picture. More severe anaemia when combined with thalassaemia.

Diagnosis: Family history and NGS or PCR demonstrating abnormal alpha globin chain length or mutation in the terminal codon of alpha gene.

Treatment: Supportive care with folic acid. Transfusions in more severe phenotypes or when combined with thalassaemia.

Sickle Cell Trials Summarised

Even though it is not crucial to quote trials in the exam, having a broad understanding of the trial in SCD is important and good for backing up your comments in an essay.

STOP trial: Stroke prevention trial in Sickle Cell Anaemia

Design: Multicentre randomised controlled blinded trial in 1995 looking at 2 groups of HbSS or HbSbeta0 children with abnormal TCD randomised to standard of care or chronic transfusion.

Primary outcomes: Reducing HbS% to < 30% by transfusion reduced the risk of first stroke by 70%.

Secondary outcomes: Periodic transfusion reduced silent infarcts.

Results: Red cell transfusion as primary prophylaxis reduced the chance of first stroke by 90%.

Adverse events: Increased risk of iron overload, transmission of BBV and alloimmunisation in the transfusion group.

STOP 2

Design: Follow on from STOP trial. Multicentred randomised controlled blinded trial of 2 groups of HbSS or HbS/beta0 children randomised to continuing transfusion or stopping after 30 months and monitoring TCD values or the presence of a stroke.

Primary outcomes: Presence of a stroke or monitoring of TCD values showing abnormal values in the group who had ceased transfusions.

Results: Halted as the cessation group demonstrated 79% who were shown to have developed abnormal TCD via doppler USS.

Adverse events: As above.

BABY HUG

Design: Multicentred randomised controlled blinded trial of 2 groups of HbSS or HbS/beta0 children randomised to HU or placebo for 2 years.

Primary outcomes: HU treatment on spleen size and kidney damage.

Results: Primary outcome not met but reduced pain, ACS, hospitalisation and transfusion need in HU group.

Adverse events: Mild to moderate myelosuppression in HU group so monitoring advised.

TAPS: The Transfusion alternatives preoperatively in Sickle Cell Disease

Design: Multicentred randomised controlled blinded trial of HbSS or HbS/beta0 scheduled for low/medium risk operations who were randomised to transfusion or no transfusion 10 days pre-op.

Primary outcomes: Clinically significant complications from randomisation to 30 days post-op.

Results: Decreased perioperative complications as well as post operative chest crisis in the transfusion group.

Adverse events: Only 1 episode of alloimmunisation in transfusion group.

TWiTCH: TCD with transfusions changing to Hydroxyurea

Design: Multicentred phase 3 randomised controlled trial looking at children with known abnormal TCD and the non-inferiority of HU vs standard of care, which was regular transfusions.

Primary outcomes: TCD and MRI assessment and HbS% after 2 years.

Results: TCD and HbS% were comparable in both arms and therefore HU deemed non-inferior. HU can be substituted for transfusion in children with abnormal TCD as a primary stroke prevention method.

Adverse events: Generally related to iron loading or chelation.

SWITCH: Stroke with transfusions changing to Hydroxyurea

Design: Multicentred phase 3 randomised controlled trial as above looking at stroke risk in those in HU and transfusion arms in children who have previously had a stroke with SCA.

Primary outcomes: Occurrence of a stroke in either arm as well as iron overload status measured by liver iron content.

Results: More strokes in the HU arm but still within non-inferior parameters. Equivalent liver iron content in each arm.

CLIMB: CRISPR-Cas9 gene editing for Sickle Cell Disease and Beta Thalassaemia

Design: Multicentred international randomised controlled trial looking at gene editing of CD34+ stem cells using CRISPR-Cas9 to target the *BCL11A* gene which is responsible for knocking down gamma globin production in SCA and transfusion dependent thalassaemia patients.

Primary outcomes: HbF > 20%, engraftment time and success, TRM, adverse events.

Results: High levels of HbF, absent occlusive episode or crisis, full engraftment in treated patients and no need for transfusion.

Adverse events: HLH in 1 individual which resolved, sepsis, consequences of ablative chemotherapy.

Anaemias

Iron Deficiency

Introduction: Iron deficiency is the leading cause of anaemia worldwide characterised by a microcytic anaemia due to reduced intake, malabsorption or increased losses, generally through bleeding.

Epidemiology: 5% of the UK population affected and more in higher risk groups such as pregnant women. 25% of pregnant woman anaemic in the UK. Iron deficiency responsible for 40–50% of anaemias worldwide.

Signs/symptoms: SOB, chest pain, lethargy, reduced exercise tolerance, dizziness, palpitations, pallor, alopecia and pica in extreme circumstances.

FBC: Microcytic, hypochromic anaemia with no other signs of cytopaenias or haemoglobinopathy.

Blood film: Anaemia with microcytosis and hypochromic red cells, some pencil cells and anisopoikilocytosis can be seen occasionally.

Diagnosis: Differing values based on BSH or NICE as well as disease state (i.e., pregnancy or CKD). Ferritin < 15 ug/L is diagnostic for all. If inflammation, then cannot use ferritin to diagnose. In this case TSAT < 16% is diagnostic.

In CKD ferritin < 100 ug/L or dialysis < 200 ug/L suggests iron deficiency.

In pregnancy depends on the trimester to diagnose anaemia as noted below.

Ferritin < 30 ug/L is diagnostic in pregnancy.

First: Hb < 110 g/L.

Second: Hb < 105 g/L.

Third: Hb < 100 g/L.

Pathophysiology: Deficient iron stores leads to ineffective haemoglobin synthesis and as a result reduced red cell production.

Tx at diagnosis? Yes, unless iron deficiency without anaemia and no symptoms but even so would suggest increasing dietary iron.

Other important work up: Dietary history, GI history, gynae history, OGD if unexplained for underlying GI occult malignancy.

First line tx options: Lifestyle changes and increasing dietary intake if possible. Oral supplementation with ferrous sulphate or fumarate. Recheck ferritin and Hb Levels 2–4 weeks after initiating treatment. If not tolerating oral iron either switch preparation or reduce dose. In CKD oral iron ineffective and IV iron infusion better for correcting levels and improving symptoms.

Second/third line: IV iron infusion based on target Hb and weight of patient. For those who are intolerant of oral iron, fail to respond or CKD. IV iron in pregnancy after second trimester for those who don't respond to oral. Consider in those who need pre-op iron supplementation but without time to wait for oral iron to work.

Important side effects of tx: GI upset with oral iron, reaction to IV iron infusion ranging from mild febrile to anaphylaxis.

Supportive care: Orange juice with tablets for enhanced absorption, laxatives or loperamide, Omeprazole if UGI symptoms bad.

Other considerations: Gynae review and consideration of norethisterone in women of childbearing age with menorrhagia. Repeat Hb testing 2–3 weeks after starting treatment, longer treatment (3 months) in pregnancy and postpartum.

Guidelines:

https://onlinelibrary.wiley.com/doi/full/10.1111/bjh.17900

https://onlinelibrary.wiley.com/doi/full/10.1111/bjh.16221

Functional Iron Deficiency

Introduction: Ineffective incorporation of iron into bone marrow erythroid precursors despite adequate iron stores reflected by ferritin or TSAT.
Epidemiology: Recognised cause of anaemia of chronic disease. Small subtype of FID which can be precipitated by ESA therapy.
Signs/symptoms: As above for anaemia, often associated with chronic disease i.e., renal, autoimmune and cancer.
FBC: MCV and MCH may be normal or low. The % of hypochromatic red cells will be low known as %HRC. Other markers which may be altered include a low Ret-he, a marker of reticulocyte haemoglobin or raised ZPP, a by-product of haem synthesis.
Blood film: Similar to IDA. May be rouleaux due to chronic inflammation.
Diagnosis: Ferritin < 100 or 200 ug/L in CKD or dialysis patients respectively. %HRC < 29 pg suggests FID in those on ESA or < 25 pg suggests classical IDA. Ret-He < 30.6 pg is used as a marker of responsiveness to ESA.
Pathophysiology: In the context of anaemia of chronic disease, iron transport is ineffective and hindered from transport into the bone marrow due to chronic inflammation leading to upregulation of the molecule hepcidin. Hepcidin degrades ferroportin, which is responsible for iron absorption from the GI tract.
Tx at diagnosis? Generally yes, as people will be symptomatic or anaemic and being investigated for the cause.
Other important work up: Rule out true IDA as well as other causes of anaemia such as dysplasia or malignancy based on film or cytopaenias.
Treatment options: Treat underlying cause. ESA weekly and IV iron as mentioned above. Tailor dose and frequency as per symptoms.
Important side effects of tx: As above for IV iron. ESA can cause VTE, hypertension or exacerbate IHD.
Other considerations: Assess response to EPO and IV iron after treatment course. Assess symptom improvement in CKD or dialysis patients.
Guidelines:
https://onlinelibrary.wiley.com/doi/full/10.1111/bjh.12311

B12 and Folate Deficiency

Introduction: Megaloblastic anaemia due to B12 or folate deficiency caused by reduced absorption/intake or increased loss characterised by a broad spectrum of symptoms including peripheral neuropathy, lethargy and glossitis.

Epidemiology: Pernicious anaemia more common in Northern Europeans and B12 and folate deficiency common in malabsorptive states.

Signs/symptoms: Symptoms of anaemia, peripheral neuropathy, unsteady gait, angular cheilitis, glossitis, cognition affected and in severe cases seizures.

Causes: GI infections, malabsorption such as pernicious anaemia or IBD, medications such as colchicine, metformin, long term PPI use, GI surgery, inadequate intake such as a vegan diet, pregnancy or rare genetic disorders, alcoholism, chronic health problems such as CKD.

FBC: Macrocytic anaemia with raised MCV and RDW. In severe cases raised LDH into the thousands. Relative reticulocytopenia.

Blood film: Megaloblastic anaemia with oval macrocytes. Often hypersegmented neutrophils with 5 or more lobes. In severe cases schistocytes and haemolytic picture. Can have pancytopenia in severe cases also.

Diagnosis:

B12: Multiple different assays available and no gold standard. Serum B12 remains first line. Second line test serum MMA. Serum HTC or homocysteine also considered as other assays, but HTC has a grey area and homocysteine reduced specificity compared to MMA.

Serum B12: < 148 qmol/l and clinical signs.

Homocysteine: Raised in B12 deficiency so > 15 umol/l considered diagnostic though this varies from lab to lab.

MMA: Raised in B12 deficiency, > 0.75 umol/l high chance of diagnosis though large lab variation. Falsely elevated in CKD.

HTC: < 0.32 qmol/l was associated with an MMA > 0.45 and moderate chance of B12 deficiency. Lab to lab variation.

Folate: *Serum folate*: < 7 nmol/l is diagnostic.

Red cell folate: Potential use if clinical suspicion and normal serum folate.

Homocysteine: > 15 umol/l can indicate deficiency.

Tx at diagnosis? Yes, if asymptomatic then increases dietary intake but in most people require B12 or folate supplementation.

Other important work up: Anti-IFAB for pernicious anaemia and more specific than GAPC antibody.

First line tx:

B12: *Neurology*: 1 mg IM alternate days for 2 weeks then assess. Reticulocyte response in 1–2 weeks. Maintenance every 8 weeks.

No neurology: 1 mg IM 3 times a week for 2 weeks then assess. Reticulocyte response in 1–2 weeks. Maintenance every 12 weeks. Treatment for most patients is lifelong.

Folate: 5 mg oral folic acid daily for 4 months. Longer in pregnancy. In severe malabsorption consider 15 mg dose. In CKD give 5 mg weekly.

Second/third line: High dose oral B12 and low dose B12 can be considered in cases where IM injection not appropriate or tolerated.

Important side effects of tx: IM B12 can cause hypokalaemia, abscess at injection sites and flushing.

Supportive care: Consider pain management in severe neuropathy as well as treating any underlying cause.

Other considerations: Replace B12 first before folate to avoid subacute combined degeneration of spinal cord, check for combined iron deficiency.

Guidelines:

https://onlinelibrary.wiley.com/doi/full/10.1111/bjh.12959
https://bnf.nice.org.uk/drugs/hydroxocobalamin/

Autoimmune Haemolytic Anaemia

Introduction: Immune mediated haemolysis due to red cell antigen recognition by IgG, IgM, IgA or a combination causing a cold, warm or mixed haemolysis leading to symptomatic anaemia. Can also occur due to components of the complement system, such as C3d.

Epidemiology: 1:100,000 per year. Higher in older population. Associated with several underlying conditions such as lymphoma, medications, atypical infection, such as hepatitis C, HIV, mycoplasma or autoimmune disease such as UC or SLE.
Warm: 65%. Cold: 30%. Mixed: 5%.

Signs/symptoms: Signs of haemolysis or anaemia, hepatosplenomegaly, underlying disorder associated like lymph nodes or infective symptoms, acrocyanosis in cold, jaundice and lethargy.

FBC: Anaemia with reticulocytosis, bilirubinaemia, reduced haptoglobin and +ve DAT. DAT tells you immune mediated and type. Other findings include +ve urine haemosiderin and raised LDH.

Blood film: Spherocytes, reticulocytes, schistocytes as well as potentially underlying cause signs such as smear cells in CLL, red cell agglutination in cold AIHA.

Diagnosis: Monospecific DAT performed for anti-IgG and C3d. If -ve perform a column agglutination method with anti-IgG, IgA, IgM and C3d all included.

Warm: DAT IgG +/- C3d which bind on warming. Antigen is often high incidence. -ve DaggT and no cold associated haemolysis

Mixed: DAT IgG + C3d which usually bind at 30°C or more. Low cold antibody titre at 4°C. Antibody is not commonly specific. DaggT may be +ve at low level antibody titre for the cold antibody.

CA: DAT -ve, antibody against anti-I with titre < 1:64 at 4°C. Thermal amplitude < 25°C. Rarely exceeds 1:256 in CA.
Red cell agglutination on film and often asymptomatic with low titre +ve DaggT.

CHAD: DAT C3d +ve. DaggT +ve. 90% anti-I antibody optimally at 4°C. Cold antibody titre > 1:64 and often > 1:500 and thermal amplitude is > 30°C. Symptoms not always present.

PCH: DAT C3d +/- IgG, DaggT -ve. Antibody usually anti-P and titre < 1:64. Thermal amplitude < 20°C. Often symptoms of cold associated haemolysis. Donath Landsteiner +ve.

Pathophysiology: Depends on the type of AIHA. Can either be antibody mediated against red cell antigens leading to direct red cell lysis or uptake in the spleen to be lysed, commonly occurs with IgG. Complement cascade activation leading to red cell lysis occurs with C3d and IgM as they can fix complement leading to intravascular haemolysis, which occurs most efficiently at 4°C hence cold induced haemolysis.

Tx at diagnosis? Yes, in warm or mixed. No if CA or mild haemolysis without symptoms and chronic. May only need supportive care.

Other important work up: Medication history, family history for enzymopathy, virology, CTNCAP or PET, haematinics, autoimmune screen, G6PD, SPEP and SFLC, good medical assessment for underlying disorder, may need BMAT to rule out LPD.

Emergency scenarios: Transfuse in severe life-threatening anaemia. IVIG at 0.5 mg/kg dose or PLEX.

First line tx options:

Warm: Prednisolone 1–2 mg/kg/ day and review in 21 days to start weaning over the next 2–3 months.

CHAD: Treatment indications include severe symptomatic anaemia, circulatory collapse or transfusion dependence. Rituximab first line.

Second/third line:

Warm, PCH or mixed: Rituximab second line if no response to steroids/relapse. MMF, ciclosporin or azathioprine third line.

CHAD: Addition of fludarabine to rituximab if clonal disorder. Splenectomy for all types if refractory or consider HSCT but rare.

Prognosis: 80% of patients respond to steroids first line in warm AIHA. 20–40% remain in remission once steroids stopped.

Important side effects of tx: Steroid side effects i.e., hyperglycaemia and insomnia. Rituximab side effects infusion reactions or TB and hepatitis B reactivation. IVIG can cause hepatitis B serology false positivity.

Supportive care: Folic acid, VTE prophylaxis, bone and gastric protection for those on steroids, keep warm for those with cold AIHA.

Other considerations: ABO, Rh and Kell matched red cells, transfuse with blood warmer in cold AIHA, pregnancy guidance similar first line treatment, second line IVIG or Azathioprine but important to involve obstetrics and infant follow up at 6 weeks postpartum.

Guidelines:

https://onlinelibrary.wiley.com/doi/full/10.1111/bjh.14478

Paroxysmal Nocturnal Haemoglobinuria

Introduction: Acquired clonal disorder of HSC due to mutation in *PIGA* gene leading to complement mediated haemolytic anaemia. This is due to the loss of cell surface proteins CD55 and CD59, which are absent following the loss of cell surface anchorage proteins.

Epidemiology: Rare disease roughly 1:100,000 prevalence. 50% of AA patients have PNH clone. Affects both men and women.

Signs/symptoms: Symptomatic haemolytic anaemia, atypical thrombosis i.e., splenic vein, abdominal pain, haemoglobinuria, jaundice and reticulocytosis.

FBC/Blood film: Haemolytic anaemia picture, may arise from AA so may have bicytopaenia/pancytopaenia. DAT -ve, raised LDH.

Diagnosis: Bone marrow for PN clone if suspicion of AA. BM or PB can be analysed by flow cytometry for absent GPI proteins CD14, 16 and 25. FLAER on white cells and absences of CD55 and 59 on red cells.

Pathophysiology: *PIGA* is responsible for the production of the cells surface anchors which attach to the surface proteins CD55 and CD59. These anchors are referred to as GPI anchors and in mutations of the *PIGA* gene causes their absence and therefore the loss of CD55 and 59. This makes red cells susceptible to complemented mediated haemolysis, as these proteins act as complement regulators, leading to anaemia and increased risk of thrombosis.

Molecular: *PIGA* mutation, gene on X chromosome. *JAK2* and *CALR* mutations also noted in PNH.

Subtypes:

Classical: Symptoms and > 50% GPI deficient cells.

Underlying BMFS: Mild haemolysis, BMFS and < 50% GPI deficient cells.

Subclinical: No haemolysis, evidence of BMFs and < 10% GPI deficient cells.

Tx at diagnosis? Depends on subtype. If classical, yes. Other subtypes may only need supportive care or treat the underlying disorder.

Other important work up: Bone marrow for AA or MDS, rule out other complement disorders or causes of haemolytic anaemia, G6PD, viral screen.

First line tx options:

Eculizumab: Monoclonal antibody blocking C5 activation and activity preventing haemolysis. 900 mg every 2 weeks. Reduces haemolysis parameters back to baseline and reduces risk of VTE in SHEPHERD study.

Ravulizumab: As above but every 2 months. Both monoclonal antibodies are IV infusions and FDA approved.

Emergency scenarios: Life threatening haemolysis or massive VTE. Consider steroids in those with severe haemolysis.

Transplant: Allograft considered in those with refractory disease or underlying severe BMFS with appropriate donor.

Prognosis: Poor prognosis: VTE as complication, progression to BMFS or leukaemia, thrombocytopaenia at diagnosis or treatment failure.

Important side effects of tx: Risk of meningococcal infections on eculizumab and vaccination recommended.

Supportive care: Refer to PNH national service, red cell transfusion, complications of haemolysis i.e., cholestasis, lifelong anticoagulation if associated thrombosis.

Trials to quote: SHEPHERD: Eculizumab in PNH improved haemolysis parameters and reduced transfusion needs.

Guidelines:
https://onlinelibrary.wiley.com/doi/full/10.1111/bjh.13853

Other Rare Anaemias

A brief overview of other rarer anaemias

Diamond-Blackfan Anaemia (DBA)

Introduction: Inherited aplastic anaemia associated with mutations to ribosomal protein genes (*RPS* or *RPL*) presenting in infancy.
Symptoms: Macrocytic, reticulocytopaenia anaemia. Associated with congenital defects of skeletal, craniofacial and cardiac systems.
Diagnosis: Autosomal dominant, *RPL/S* mutations in 60% via NGS, family history in 20% though most sporadic, elevated HbF and EPO.
Treatment: Prednisolone 1 mg/kg. 70% respond. Aim to wean, though many may need chronic treatment. Transfusion program. HSCT if suitable.

Fanconi's Anaemia (FA)

Introduction: Inherited anaemia due to molecular mutation which affects all cells in the body characterised by increased chromosomal breakage.
Symptoms: Gradual pancytopenia in childhood, median age 9. Skin pigmentation, skeletal defects and developmental delay.
Diagnosis: Autosomal recessive pattern, affecting *FANC* genes. X-linked subtype rare. Increased chromosomal breakage. Increased risk of AML.
Treatment: Supportive care and transfusion, G-CSF for neutropaenia, androgen therapy, HSCT in those with suitable donor.

Congenital Dyserythropoietic Anaemia (CDA)

Introduction: Disorder of vesicle trafficking and nuclear proteins affecting children and adolescents leading to defective erythropoiesis.
Symptoms: Anaemia with iron overload symptoms, structural disorders of distal limb, hepatosplenomegaly or blindness.
Diagnosis: Autosomal recessive. Molecular shows mutations in genes such as *CDAN1* or *GATA1*. Diagnosis made by bone marrow and NGS. 3 different subtypes.
CDA 1: Macrocytic severe anaemia.
CDA 2: Variable phenotype, normocytic anaemia with associated jaundice, most common.
CDA 3: Rarest, seen in 2 families predominantly, characteristic *GATA1* mutation, anaemia and visual disturbances.
Treatment: Iron chelation and transfusion, interferon for those with more severe disease. HSCT rarely needed.

Inherited Sideroblastic Anaemia

Introduction: Disorder of haem synthesis affecting children and adolescents leading to anaemia and ring sideroblasts in the BM.

Symptoms: Symptoms of iron overload and anaemia. Rarely clinical signs or symptoms specific to disorder.

Diagnosis: X-linked or autosomal recessive. BMA showing ring sideroblasts. Associated molecular mutation such as *HSPA9* or *GLRX5*.

Treatment: Supportive care with transfusions and iron chelation. HSCT rarely needed.

Dyskeratosis Congenita

Introduction: Inherited anaemia characterised by abnormal skin pigmentation, bone marrow failure and dystrophic nails affecting adolescents.

Symptoms: As above + mucous membrane pathology, increased chromosome breakage as per FA, short telomeres, 10% risk of malignancy.

Diagnosis: X-linked, autosomal dominant and recessive forms all exist. Multiple molecular mutations recognised i.e., *TERC* or *TERT*.

Treatment: Supportive care with transfusion, trial of G-CSF or EPO, HSCT though outcomes often poor.

Schwann-Diamond Syndrome

Introduction: BM failure disorder affecting GI and endocrine system presenting in childhood.

Symptoms: Diarrhoea, pancreatic insufficiency, developmental delay, neutropaenia and anaemia. 25% chance of AML development.

Diagnosis: Autosomal recessive with molecular mutations in *SBDS*.

Treatment: Supportive care with GCSF and pancreatic hormones such as Creon. HSCT if suitable.

Red Cell Enzymopathies and Membranopathies

G6PD Deficiency

Introduction: Deficiency in the enzyme G6PD leading to profound red cell haemolysis due to oxidative stress from environmental triggers.

Epidemiology: 200+ molecular mutations, affects more than 400 million people. More common in Africa, India, Southeast Asia or Mediterranean.

Signs/symptoms: Jaundice, symptomatic anaemia, haemoglobinuria, associated with other red cell disorders i.e., HbSS.

FBC/Blood film: Haemolytic anaemia with "Ghost cells" suggesting oxidative stress, schistocytes and spherocytes also likely seen. Heinz bodies and reticulocytosis, raised LDH and bilirubin, DAT -ve.

Diagnosis: Screening done on clinical ground or those who may need drugs which exacerbate i.e., Rasburicase in those high risk of TLS.

Screening: Fluorescent spot or dye discoloration assay in males but not in females. Females should measure activity via quantitative spectrophotometric assay. Males should have quantitative assay only to confirm if screening assays are abnormal.

Molecular: Consider if results are borderline, females or males with Klinefelter's syndrome.

Pathophysiology: G6PD is present in all cells but in RBC is vital for NADPH production as the first step in the pentose phosphate shunt. Production of NADPH allows for red cell glutathione to be in its reduced state and should oxidative stress occur it can deal with it. In G6PD deficiency this glutathione state does not occur so that when oxidative stress occurs following a trigger widespread haemolysis ensues. Mutations occur on X chromosome so the phenotype much more severe in males than females.

Tx at diagnosis? No, but avoid certain drugs such as antimalarial, antibiotics, anaesthesia, rasburicase and many more.

Other important work up: Rule out other causes of immune and non-immune haemolysis, viral infections, mechanical haemolysis.

First line tx options: In severe haemolysis transfuse and consider red cell exchange if life threatening or in young.

Important side effects of tx: Risk associated with chronic transfusion as mentioned previously.

Supportive care: IVF during haemolytic episodes, folic acid, avoiding drugs which cause haemolysis.

Other considerations: Unreliable G6PD assay after transfusion or severe haemolysis, elevated WCC can falsely elevate G6PD levels.

Guidelines:

https://onlinelibrary.wiley.com/doi/10.1111/bjh.16366

PK Deficiency

Introduction: Inherited disorder associated with deficiency or absence of the enzyme pyruvate kinase leading to a haemolytic anaemia.

Epidemiology: Rare disorder. Variable prevalence reported from 1:20,000–1,000,000.

Signs/symptoms: Variable based on inheritance, haemolytic anaemia, occasionally splenomegaly and jaundice. Patient may need splenectomy or cholecystectomy in severe haemolysis. Other complications include osteoporosis, iron overload, aplastic crisis and pulmonary hypertension.

FBC/Blood film: Reticulocytosis with spherocyte, Heinz bodies, schistocytes, target cells if hyposplenism, raised LDH and DAT -ve.

Diagnosis: Measurement of PK activity in red cells or molecular mutation in *PKLR* gene. Family history often present.

Pathophysiology: Autosomal recessive condition due to mutations in the *PKLR* gene. This mutation prevents ATP formation at the last step of the glycolysis cycle preventing pyruvate formation and reducing the red cell life span from 4 months to 1–2 weeks. Unlike G6PD where there are triggers causing severe haemolysis PK deficiency leads to chronic low-level haemolysis constantly but can be exacerbated by causes such as infections or medications.

Tx at diagnosis? Yes, with supportive care. Treatment to stop haemolysis is rarely needed.

Other important work up: As above for ruling out other causes of haemolysis.

First line tx options: Generally supportive care is all that's needed and avoiding triggers.

Mitapivat: Oral activator of PK which has been approved by the FDA if needed.

Supportive care: Folic acid, transfusion in severe anaemia, splenectomy can be done though rare, iron chelation in those having chronic transfusion, managing high blood pressure, managing cholestasis.

Other considerations: Monitor for viral infections, can develop aplastic crisis in parvovirus B19 infection.

Hereditary Spherocytosis

Introduction: Inherited red cell membrane disorder affecting cytoskeletal proteins causing a spherocytosis with a spectrum of symptoms.

Epidemiology: Diagnosis made in childhood if symptomatic or at routine health checks later in life if not i.e., booking appointments, GP registration etc. Relatively common with 1:2,000–5,000 Northern Europeans affected.

Signs/symptoms: Jaundice, anaemia, splenomegaly, reticulocytosis, symptoms of chronic haemolysis i.e., cholestasis. Spectrum of symptoms from none to severe haemolysis.

FBC/Blood film: Anaemia, reticulocytosis, spherocytosis, DAT -ve, elevated LDH and bilirubin.

Diagnosis: Combination of clinical history, family history and laboratory investigations. Recommended tests when no family history or if asymptomatic are the EMA binding test and NGS. If family history with offspring or sibling affected with symptoms and characteristic film and lab criteria, generally the additional diagnostic tests are not needed. Osmotic fragility no longer recommended.

EMA binding: Flow cytometry assay. EMA binds to specific transmembrane proteins so if they are mutated or absent florescence is reduced.

Cryohaemolysis: Increased lysis observed in HS as cells are more susceptible to cold conditions than normal healthy red cells.

Pathophysiology: Generally autosomal dominant inheritance. Mutations in α or β spectrin, ankyrin, band 3 or protein 4.2 can occur on their own or in combination. This impacts the red cell shape and size by loss of the membrane integrity which leads to reduced life span and splenomegaly.

Molecular: Molecular mutations that occur in above proteins are *SPTA1*, *SPTB*, *ANK1*, *SLC4A1* or *EPB42* respectively.

Classification: Based on Hb, reticulocytes, bilirubin, spectrin molecules per erythrocyte and determines whether splenectomy may be recommended. Those with moderate disease or worse (moderate anaemia, raised reticulocytes and bilirubin with spectrin molecules 50%) and transfusion dependent may need splenectomy.

Tx at diagnosis? Unless symptomatic no. But provide supportive care with folic acid and regular haem follow up for all.

Other important work up: Haemoglobinopathy screen, rule out acquired haemolysis i.e., AIHA, drugs or viral.

Treatment options: Transfusion in those who are moderately to severely symptomatic.

Splenectomy: If moderate/severe disease, causing significant symptoms to impair quality of life or if transfusion dependent. Laparoscopic associated with better post-op recovery. In children perform cholecystectomy at same time if symptomatic cholestasis. Ideally perform splenectomy after the age of 6 and before 12.

Emergency scenarios: Severe neonatal jaundice. Treatment is red cell exchange. Aplastic crisis or ruptured spleen can also occur

Important side effects of tx: Risk of chronic transfusion. Risk of sepsis or atypical infections following splenectomy.

Supportive care: Folate therapy and under the care of haem even if well for annual follow up, penicillin V and vaccinations in splenectomy cases.

Other considerations: Co-inheritance of other red cell disorders such as haemo-globinopathy can delay diagnosis or make phenotype worse, testing after 6 months of age if baby well to assess film morphology more accurately, monitor for aplastic crisis or extramedullary haematopoiesis, genetic counselling. DEXA scan for osteoporosis and ECHO for pulmonary hypertension.

Guidelines:

https://onlinelibrary.wiley.com/doi/full/10.1111/j.1365-2141.2011.08921.x

Hereditary/SE Asian Ovalocytosis

Introduction: Inherited red cell disorder primarily affecting Southeast Asian population due to cytoskeletal mutations causing oval shaped erythrocytes.

Epidemiology: More common in Southeast Asian populations and rare in Europe. More common in malaria endemic areas.

Signs/symptoms: Generally asymptomatic. Neonatal jaundice, signs and symptoms of haemolytic anaemia as above, mild splenomegaly and cholestasis compared to HS, symptoms often disappear later in life or become milder.

FBC/Blood film: Macrocytic ovalocytes, generally > 25%. Mild haemolytic picture, DAT -ve, stomatocytes seen occasionally.

Diagnosis: Often a family history. Combination of family history, clinical symptoms and molecular showing abnormality in gene coding for band 3 protein. EMA dye binding will be low.

Pathophysiology: Band 3 protein is a crucial anion exchange at the red cell membrane. When mutated the cell stability is compromised due to ineffective anion transportation and changes in pH leading to red cell lysis. Mutations in the protein also affects other cytoskeletal proteins. Homozygous mutations often incompatible with life.

Molecular: Heterogenous mutations affecting *SLC4A1* gene on chromosome 17 which codes for band 3 protein.

Tx at diagnosis? No, unless symptomatic with haemolytic anaemia.

Other important work up: As above for ruling out acquired haemolysis or other co-existing haemoglobinopathies or membranopathies.

First line tx options: Supportive care with folic acid. Splenectomy in severe phenotype with symptomatic splenomegaly or transfusion dependence though this is very rare. Commonly patients are largely asymptomatic.

Emergency scenarios: Severe neonatal jaundice. Treatment is red cell exchange. Aplastic crisis can present following infection though rare.

Hereditary Elliptocytosis

Introduction: Inherited red cell disorder due to mutations in spectrin or band protein 4.1 leading to elliptocytes and variable phenotypes.

Epidemiology: More common in malaria endemic areas. 1:2,000–5,000 Europeans. Generally autosomal dominant inheritance.

Signs/symptoms: Spectrum of symptoms including symptoms of haemolytic anaemia and splenomegaly. Most asymptomatic.

FBC/Blood film: Signs of haemolytic anaemia with elliptocytes, mild chronic haemolysis, DAT -ve, reticulocytosis and raised LDH.

Diagnosis: Made by family history and characteristic blood film changes. Molecular screening reveals mutations in the below affected genes.

Pathophysiology: Mutations in the mentioned genes which affect the scaffolding proteins leads to loss of elastic recoil in the red cell membrane and characteristic elliptocyte shape and shortened red cell lifespan.

Molecular: Heterogenous mutations affecting *SPTA1*, *SPTB* or *EPB41* which affects α or β spectrin and protein 4.1 respectively.

Tx at diagnosis? No, unless severe haemolysis and symptomatic anaemia. Supportive care with folic acid for all.

Other important work up: As above for ruling out acquired haemolysis or other co-existing haemoglobinopathies or membranopathies.

First line tx options: Generally, just supportive care, transfusion in severe anaemia or exchange in neonates with haemolysis though this is rare. Splenectomy rarely needed but can be considered on case-by-case basis i.e., homozygous with severe haemolysis and symptoms of splenomegaly impacting quality of life.

Supportive care: Folic acid and antibiotic prophylaxis for those who do have splenectomy.

Other considerations: As above for all membranopathies.

Guidelines:
https://onlinelibrary.wiley.com/doi/10.1111/bjh.18191

Hereditary Haemochromatosis

Introduction: Disorder of iron absorption due to various molecular mutations leading to organ damage. Multiple different molecular subtypes that have various phenotypes which impact the management of the disease.

Epidemiology: Common in Northern Europeans affecting 1:200–500, compared to the rest of the world where it is less prevalent.

Signs/symptoms: May be asymptomatic or have family history, picked up on screening tests or well person test. Those with symptoms vary with homozygous worse than heterozygous. New diabetes, liver dysfunction, erectile dysfunction, cardiac failure. Any tissue can be damaged. Women often present later than men due to iron loss through menstruation.

Bloods: Often normal FBC and film. Raised ferritin or TSAT or both. Signs of organ infiltration i.e., deranged LFTs or raised BNP.

Diagnosis:

Bloods: All should get FBC, ferritin, TSAT but check on fasting sample as elevated following recent intake of iron, LFTs. Ferritin > 1,000 ug/l and deranged LFTs then refer to hepatologist. Ferritin > 200 ug/l and TSAT > 40% in Women and > 300 ug/l and TSAT > 50% in men should have molecular testing. If patient well and only ferritin raised without TSAT exclude reactive causes. If no reactive cause and ferritin > 1000 ug/L, then either follow up in 3–6 months if asymptomatic or MRI liver if unwell to assess iron overload status.

Molecular: Perform if above criteria met or family history. *C282Y* and *H63D* performed. Extended panel can be done for rarer genotypes.

Pathophysiology: Mutations in the *HFE* gene leads to reduced hepcidin expression in macrophages of the reticuloendothelial system which are the main component of iron storage. Hepcidin would usually prevent excess iron absorption through the GI tract by inhibiting ferroportin. When hepcidin is down regulated, as is the case in hemochromatosis, the absorption from the GI tract is not regulated and once the RES macrophages are saturated the left-over absorbed iron is deposited in the cells of tissues leading to symptoms.

Molecular: Most commonly due to autosomal recessive inheritance with mutations of the *HFE* gene on chromosome 6.

Tx at diagnosis? With nearly all subtypes yes, except heterozygous *C282Y* may only require monitoring. Yes, in *C282Y* homozygous or *C282Y/H63D* if associated with other co-morbidities like alcohol excess or diabetes etc but if on its own then generally just monitoring. Monitoring only in *H63D* homozygous. *H63D* and *C282Y* carrier states don't require any monitoring.

Other important work up: Rule out reactive causes, monitor AFP in clinic for associated risk of HCC.

Subtypes:

Type 1: *C282Y* or *H63D* mutations. Later associated with worse iron loading.

Type 2: Juvenile form affecting *HFE2* or *HAMP* genes. Severe iron loading and cardiac failure can readily occur. Presenting in young patients.

Type 3: Transferrin receptor 2 deficiency due to mutation in the *TFR2* gene. Iron loading severity in between type 1 and 2.

Type 4: Rare variant with autosomal recessive inheritance affecting *SLC40A1* encoding for ferroportin. Severity of iron loading is only very mild. 4A is mild whereas 4B is similar in phenotype to type 1.

Type 5: Rare autosomal dominant type described in 1 Japanese family affecting *FTH1* gene.

Imaging: Ferriscan or liver MRI in those with elevated LFTs. Ferriscan not readily available at all places so MRI if not. USS liver as back up.

First line tx options:

Induction: Weekly venesection aiming for ferritin < 30 ug/l and TSAT < 50%. Monitor FBC.

Maintenance: Aim serum ferritin < 50 ug/l and TSAT < 50%. Everyone different but often every 2–3 months. Depends on phenotype. Consider blood donation and annual monitoring with normal iron parameters. Not suitable in cirrhotic patients. Cirrhotic patients should have 6 monthly liver USS and AFP to screen for risk of HCC.

Prognosis: Worse outcomes in those with cirrhosis or diabetes. Once cirrhotic then there is a significantly increased chance of HCC.

Important side effects of tx: Anaemia from venesection, monitor FBC regularly.

Supportive care: Diabetic medications, pain relief and physio for arthropathy, diuretics for CCF though can be reversible once iron loading is resolved via venesection, endocrine review for pituitary iron loading causing hormonal problems.

Trials to quote: HEIRS: Assessing the prevalence of *C282Y* showed more common in white Northern Europeans.

Other considerations: HCC risk, MDT for diabetic input or other specialities, clinical psychologist and genetic counselling, liver biopsy in those with ferritin > 1,000 ug/l and deranged LFTs to assess fibrosis. Perform TSAT fasted to get accurate result.

Guidelines:

https://onlinelibrary.wiley.com/doi/full/10.1111/bjh.15166
https://onlinelibrary.wiley.com/doi/pdf/10.1111/bjh.15164

Immune Thrombocytopaenia Purpura

Introduction: Isolated thrombocytopaenia, often immune mediated leading to increased platelet destruction and reduced production.

Epidemiology: Incidence 5:100,000, slightly less in childhood. Most children require no treatment (85%). Slight female predominance.

Signs/symptoms: Asymptomatic in many, petechial rash or bruising, bleeding typically mucosal but in severe can be intraabdominal or intracranial. Generally spontaneous bleeding does not occur when platelets are greater than 30×10^9/L.

FBC/Blood film: Isolated thrombocytopaenia varying in severity, exclude TTP looking for fragments. <u>Severe</u>: Platelets < 30.

Risk factors: Pregnancy, auto-immune disease, infection, vaccination, malignancy, medications, more common in women of childbearing age.

Diagnosis: Diagnosis of exclusion. Bone marrow only recommended where neoplasm suspected, 60 or older, considering splenectomy or in relapsed ITP. Anti-platelet antibodies not advised except in certain cases i.e., refractory, drug-induced or distinguishing between MDS and ITP.

Pathophysiology: Primary hypothesis is the reaction of T-helper cells with APC in the spleen presenting platelet proteins to T-helper cells leading to B-cell antibody production and cytotoxic T-cell responses against platelets in the peripheral blood and spleen. Also, evidence that immune mediated inhibition of megakaryocyte in the bone marrow by B and T-cells reducing platelet production.

Tx at diagnosis? Depends on severity, bleeding phenotype and clinical scenario i.e., surgery. Asymptomatic and platelets < 30 then treat unless reason not to.

Other important work up: Good clinical history using BAT and rule out MDS or leukaemia, viral bloods, *H. Pylori*, liver screen, drug history, TFT, autoimmune screen, USS abdomen, lymphocyte subsets, rule out acute infection, check film for no platelet clumping and if so do citrated sample, rule out type 2b VWD or platelet function disorder, DAT and Immunoglobulin levels, APS screen and autoimmune screen for disorders such as SLE.

First line tx options:

<u>Prednisolone</u>: 1 mg/kg OD for 2–4 weeks and then taper 5–10 mg/week and monitor platelets. If no response after 1 month, then rapid taper and move onto second line. Safe in pregnancy as is IVIG.

<u>IVIG</u>: Good for elevating platelet count initially if bleeding symptoms or pre-surgery but not durable. Dose of 0.4 g/kg/day for 5/7 or 1 g/kg for 2 days. Repeated up to 7 days later with another 1 g/kg if no response.

TPO-RA: Good efficacy in splenectomised and not. Easy to administer. Romiplostim S/C, Eltrombopag PO. Titrate based on count. Approved to be given first line following COVID-19 era or as second line. Good responses with long term durable response in 20–30%. Avatrombopag also now NICE approved for refractory ITP as an oral agent.

Platelet targets (× 10⁹/L):

Tooth extraction: ≥ 30.

Minor surgery: ≥ 30.

Vaginal delivery or C-section: ≥ 50.

Major surgery or LP: ≥ 80.

ICB: ≥ 100.

Emergency scenarios: ICB or life-threatening bleeding: IVIG +/- high dose steroids and platelet transfusion. TXA also.

Second Line: Consider a trial as well as at diagnosis. Considered chronic refractory ITP when failing first and second-line therapy.

High dose steroid: Consider dexamethasone or methylprednisolone if responded before +/- a new line of therapy.

Rituximab: Often used second or third line. Many respond and often for > 9 months but relapse rates high.

MMF: 50% response rate and easy for patient as a tablet and well tolerated. Response takes 1–2 months and risk of infection or cytopaenias.

Third line onwards:

AZA or ciclosporin: Slow acting. Can be given with other agents i.e., steroids. Around 50% will respond.

Dapsone: Around 50% respond though not sustained for long. Poor response rates post-splenectomy.

Alemtuzumab: Good ORR and often durable lasting more than 4 months. Risk of neutropaenia or reactions so need careful monitoring.

Vincristine: Potential for a role in splenectomised patient with 65% responding but durability not good with < 10% sustaining response.

Anti-D: Not often used but good ORR in 70–90%. Lasts around a month in 50%. Don't use post-splenectomy or if refractory.

Danazol: Consider in those with autoimmune disorder driving ITP. Use as steroid sparing agent. 60% respond lasting > 2 months.

Splenectomy: Good CR rates but complications associated with procedure and risk of infections afterwards.

Others: SYK or BTK inhibitors such as fostamatinib or rilzabrutinib also available and NICE approved

Prognosis: Long term remission in 10–20% following steroids. High ORR in IVIG though responses only last around a month.

Important side effects of tx:

Bone protection: Lifestyle advice for all on steroids +/- vitamin D and calcium supplements. FRAX assessment for risk of fracture. All high risk should receive bisphosphonate or alternative for bone protection. Cumulative dose of steroid is often around 1–2 g total.

TPO-RA: Risk of thrombosis or leukoerythroblastic film due to stimulation of marrow.

Supportive care: Platelet transfusion only in ICB or life-threatening bleeding, vaccinations and penicillin V in splenectomy patients, TXA in bleeding, factor VIIa in severe bleeding episodes, MDT approach with obstetrics and considerations to help menorrhagia i.e., norethisterone.

Other considerations: Steroid card or ITP card, emergency TXA at home, safety netting if trauma, education on risk factor or triggers, cord platelet counts and may need to treat neonate in obstetrics, LMWH in those post-op/postpartum once stable counts, add patient to ITP registry.

Guidelines:

https://onlinelibrary.wiley.com/doi/10.1046/j.1365-2141.2003.04131.x

https://ashpublications.org/bloodadvances/article/3/23/3829/429213/American-Society-of-Hematology-2019-guidelines-for

Thrombotic Thrombocytopaenia Purpura

Introduction: Life-threatening acquired or congenital disorder due to deficiency in ADAMTS13 leading to thrombosis, bleeding, MAHA, fever, renal dysfunction, and neurological complications. Congenital TTP is rare and affects the *ADAMTS13* gene causing < 5% activity.

Epidemiology: Rare disorder with incidence of 1:200,000. Risk factors include pregnancy, HIV infection, malignancy especially adenocarcinomas, post-transplant, pancreatitis and medications i.e., quinine, chemotherapy and COCP.

Signs/symptoms: Fever, neurological symptoms such as headache, visual or speech disturbance or seizures, jaundice, abdominal or chest pain.

FBC/Blood film: Thrombocytopaenia, schistocytes with > 5 per HPF, anaemia, reticulocytosis, DAT -ve, raised LDH.

Diagnosis: Clinical manifestations + blood film findings + ADAMTS13 assay looking at activity, antigen and inhibitor. ADMATS13 < 5 IU/dL and IgG antibody or inhibitor is diagnostic.

Pathophysiology: ADAMTS13 cleaves VWF in normal physiology. In TTP either due to antibody formation (acquired) or deficiency (congenital). ADAMTS13 is deficient and VWF is not cleaved allowing ultra large weight multimers to form which would not normally. These multimers accumulate and unfurl in vessels where there are high shear stress rates, such as the microvasculature, cause platelet aggregation and thrombosis.

Molecular: In congenital TTP mutations in the *ADAMTS13* gene.

Tx at diagnosis? YES! Do not wait for ADAMTS13 to start PLEX if suspected. Start within 4–8 hours and treat as medical emergency. Transfer to recognised TTP centre urgently. If not possible then start treatment but transfer is crucial for ongoing treatment and best outcome.

Other important work up: Drug history, pregnancy test, rule out infection, autoimmune screen, vasculitis screen, APS screen, CTNCAP to rule out malignancy, check BP, CVC line and anaesthetic support, troponin, Urine PCR, stool culture for *E. coli* 0157, amylase, viral screen.

First line tx options:

<u>PLEX</u>: OctaplasLG 1.5 plasma volumes TDS and then 1 plasma volume OD. PLEX should carry on for 2 days post-platelet count remaining > 150×10^9/L. Use S/D plasma infusion or factor VIII in congenital TTP. Not indicated in post-BMT or malignancy associated.

<u>Steroids</u>: Methylprednisolone 1 g OD or prednisolone 1 mg/kg/day for 3 days.

<u>Caplacizumab</u>: 10 mg IV before PLEX and then 10 mg S/C after each PLEX and for 30 days after finishing. Reduces PLEX days.

<u>Rituximab</u>: In treatment resistant HIV associated TTP or if there is cardiac or neurological involvement.

<u>HAART</u>: In HIV associated TTP with PLEX and continue after TTP remission.

Second/third line: Always consider clinical trial, even at diagnosis. Increased PLEX frequency if relapsing disease. Splenectomy rare.

Rituximab: Can delay the incidence of relapse if used during acute episode.

Ciclosporin: Good responses but around 1/3 will relapse after stopping treatment.

Prognosis: Untreated mortality is 90%. Most deaths occur within 1 day of presentation. Worse outcomes in neurological or cardiac symptoms. Relapse occurs in around 35% of cases with an episode of TTP > 30 days since remission defining relapse. Lifelong follow up with ADAMTS13 monitoring and neurology and psychology support. Give rituximab pre-emptively if ADAMTS13 levels fall below 20 IU/dL.

Important side effects of tx:

PLEX: Hypotension, CVC line risks, hypocalcaemia. Steroids side effects mentioned previously.

Rituximab: TB or Hep B reactivation.

Caplacizumab: Increased bleeding risk and contraindicated in bleeding.

Supportive care: PPI, folic acid, bone protection for steroid use, LMWH and aspirin once platelet count > 50 × 10^9/L, red cell transfusion if needed, platelet transfusion contraindicated unless life threatening bleeding, regular monitoring of ADAMTS13 levels.

Trials to quote: HERCULES and TITAN: Caplacizumab and PLEX vs placebo and PLEX. Reduced time to platelet recovery and PLEX days when Caplacizumab given.

Other considerations: ADAMTS13 often not done on site if in small hospital, MDT approach for pregnancy associated, ITU support, TTP card, counsel patients on risk of relapse and symptoms to look out for.

Guidelines:

https://onlinelibrary.wiley.com/doi/full/10.1111/bjh.19026

Haemolytic Uraemic Syndrome

Introduction: Acquired disorder characterised by thrombocytopaenia, fever, renal failure and MAHA. 2 distinct subtypes referred to as diarrhoea +ve and atypical HUS. Diarrhoea +ve associated with *E. coli* 0157 infection.

Epidemiology: Atypical HUS is very rare with incidence roughly 1:500,000. 70% of atypical HUS have underlying molecular mutation.

Signs/symptoms: Symptoms of haemolytic anaemia, diarrhoea, abdominal pain, associated with genetic and acquired disorders of complement, HIV or malignancy, autoimmune disease such as SLE, pregnancy or medications such as chemotherapy. No neurological signs but renal dysfunction severe which can lead to AKI requiring dialysis.

FBC/Blood film: Similar to TTP and often hard to distinguish.

Diagnosis: Often hard to distinguish from TTP but generally ADAMTS13 activity normal in atypical HUS and certainly not < 5% as seen in TTP. Diarrhoea requires +ve associated infection i.e., *E. coli* 0157. Renal dysfunction which occurs in atypical HUS is much worse than in TTP. Flow cytometry on PB shows reduced CD46 expression on white cells. Molecular panel showing characteristic mutations.

Pathophysiology/Molecular: Mutations in genes affecting complement regulation such as *CFH*, *CFI*, *CFD*, *CFHR15*, *C3* and CD46 in atypical HUS leading to uncontrolled complement activation via the alternative pathway.

Tx at diagnosis? YES! Without treatment high mortality and risk of CKD + dialysis long term.

Other important work up: Complement levels, factor H and I and antibodies against complement, molecular panel on PB for associated mutations, stool, and blood cultures, CTNCAP for malignancy, ADAMTS13 to rule out TTP

First line tx options: Always consider clinical trials up front.

PLEX: 1–2 plasma volumes and assess clinically and biochemically responses.

Eculizumab: Use as first line alongside PLEX or alone. Improved mortality and morbidity. Lifelong prophylaxis recommended in those receiving a kidney transplant.

Transplant: Consider liver and kidney transplant in those with atypical HUS and *CFH* or *CFI* molecular mutations.

Prognosis: 25% mortality in all atypical HUS and 50% don't recover renal function completely.

Important side effects of tx: As above for TTP treatments. Vaccination against meningococcal infections in Eculizumab.

Supportive care: MDT with renal, transfusion if needed, folic acid, LMWH, avoid platelet transfusion unless life threatening bleeding, CVC.

Guidelines:
https://onlinelibrary.wiley.com/doi/full/10.1111/j.1365-2141.2009.07916.x
https://onlinelibrary.wiley.com/doi/full/10.1111/j.1365-2141.2012.09167.x

Red Cell Lab Principles

Sickle Cell Solubility Test

Introduction: Assay to show the presence of HbS following the addition of a reducing agent to precipitate the abnormal haemoglobin.
What it measures: The presence of HbS.
How to perform:
1. Sample collected via venepuncture.
2. Whole blood sample has reducing agent added, such as sodium hydrosulphite, and the red cells are lysed releasing Hb molecule.
3. HbS precipitates whereas HbA dissolves in plasma.

Results interpretation: Presence of HbS leads to turbid appearance whereas HbA in solution is clear.
Benefits: High sensitivity and specificity for HbS, easy to perform with widely available agents, cheap.
Limitations: False -ve in patients with anaemia, transfusion neonates or HPFH. False +ve in hyperviscosity. Result interpreted by person so subjective nature if borderline results. Doesn't differentiate between trait and disease.

Haemoglobin Electrophoresis

Introduction: Assay performed to differentiate between various haemoglobin molecules based on their molecular charge.

What it measures: Various haemoglobin molecules such as HbA, HbS, HbF, HbC and HbE. Can diagnose haemoglobinopathy or thalassaemia.

How to perform:

1. Sample collected via venepuncture and hemolysate is prepared from the sample.
2. Sample is added to electrophoresis starch gel and attached to power supply in liquid support medium.
3. Power turned on and the haemoglobin molecules migrate at different rates forming various bands based on charge and weight.
4. Comparison of electrophoresis pattern compared to healthy controls and known disease.
5. Haemoglobin can be quantified thereafter by elution and spectrophotometry.

Results interpretation: Abnormal haemoglobins are detected and quantified which can form a diagnosis based on patterns seen in certain haemoglobinopathies. i.e., HbSS disease shows HbS% of 90% etc.

Benefits: Gives a diagnosis most of the time as relatively cheap.

Limitations: False -ve if recent transfusion. HbF is alkali so cannot be quantified by this method. More time consuming than sickle cell solubility and relies on expert interpretation.

High Performance Liquid Chromatography

Introduction: Assay which separates compounds in a lysate based on the different polarity which can then be separated based on light absorbance of each component, in this case different haemoglobin molecules.

What it measures: The absorbance of light from different eluates flowing precipitation based on their polarity.

How to perform:

1. Collect sample via venepuncture and prepare for the injector system as per the manufacturer's specifications.
2. Load sample into the column and it is passed through the column at a set flow rate by pressurised pump.
3. Column containing small absorbent silica beads are separated as the sample is pushed through the column based on varying polarity. The non-polar molecules pass through and the highly polar ones are absorbed by the silica beads.
4. The separated eluates are then passed through an LED system where light absorbance is detected by a detector and plots peaks of difference.

Results interpretation: Different peaks on the chromatograph correspond to different haemoglobin molecules and disease.

Benefits: Accurate and can assay multiple Hb molecules in complex haemoglobinopathies, checks for HbF, gives diagnosis.

Limitations: Expensive, time consuming, needs specialist equipment, lab staff and lab.

Heinz Body Preparation

Introduction: An assay performed looking for inclusions within the red cell which are denatured haemoglobin seen in haemolytic anaemia, oxidative stress, haemoglobinopathies or splenectomy/hyposplenism.

What it measures: The presence of denatured haemoglobin.

How to perform:

1. Whole blood is collected in a tube with anticoagulant via venepuncture and used for the assay.
2. Add 1 ml of blood to 4 ml of methyl violet solution and leave to stand for 10 minutes at room temperature.
3. Add the prepared solution to a slide and view under the microscope looking for the red cell inclusions, known as Heinz Bodies.

Results interpretation: The presence of Heinz bodies should point towards one of the conditions mentioned above.

Benefits: Helps to diagnose intrinsic red cell pathology, cheap, easy for lab staff to perform, can be done at most labs.

Limitations: Does not provide diagnosis, relies on lab staff preparation and time, variation based on different reagents in lab and across labs.

Haematological Oncology

The haematological oncology section is probably the most familiar section for all of us given that we will have all likely managed these conditions both as inpatients and outpatients. This field is constantly evolving with new treatments being licensed regularly meaning we must constantly update our knowledge. Immunophenotyping panels and molecular markers can also cause quite a headache for exam candidates when revising.

Even though I have whittled down the information in this section to all the necessary things you need to know, it is still the longest and most detailed in the book. For a more comprehensive overview of this section, refer to the guidelines or the new WHO classification of myeloid and lymphoid neoplasms as well as good practice papers. My experience of revising this topic is straightforward: you get out what you put in, and the more you read around the subject, the more rounded and deeper the understanding of it. As well as using this book there are some great podcasts about updates and general management of these conditions.

My final tip: if you work up a patient with a new diagnosis, read the section on that diagnosis the evening after. Not only will it consolidate your learning, but it will make you a better haematologist. I found this useful for signposting in my mind when revising a topic. For example, "I remember doing the marrow on Mrs Jones who had poor risk AML because she was *FLT3* mutated and *NPM1* wild type and because of that she needed standard DA + the *FLT3* inhibitor Gilteritinib and then went on to have an allograft in CR1". This sticks with you much better than randomly diving into topics willy-nilly!

Lymphomas

B-Cell Lymphomas

While writing this section the WHO 2022 updates were published halfway through. Overleaf is a table of some of the key updates relevant to the book in terms of new terminology for the B-cell Lymphomas. Often the phrasing of the disorder has been changed slightly or new classifications are added. Many of the new additions are very rare and further reading should be sought, if interested. I have tried to incorporate the new classifications and terminology though for the exam I suspect the older definitions would not be marked negatively if mentioned. There are multiple articles and reviews detailing all changes online.

WHO 2022 update	WHO 2017 classification
In-situ follicular B-cell neoplasm	In-situ follicular neoplasia
In-situ mantle cell neoplasm	In-situ mantle cell neoplasia
DLBCL/high grade B-cell lymphoma with MYC/BCL2 or BCL6 rearrangements	High grade B-cell lymphoma with MYC/BCL2 or BCL6 rearrangements
High grade B-cell lymphoma with 11q aberrations	Burkitt-like lymphoma with 11q aberration
EBV +ve DLBCL	EBV +ve DLBCL, NOS
Mediastinal grey zone lymphoma	B-cell lymphoma, unclassifiable, with features intermediate between DLBCL and classic Hodgkin lymphoma
KSHV/HHV8 +ve DLBCL, NOS	HHV8 +ve DLBCL, NOS
KSHV/HHV8 +ve germinotrophic LPD	HHV8 +ve germinotrophic LPD
Inborn errors of immune associated lymphoid proliferation and lymphomas	LPD associated with immune disorders
Splenic B-cell lymphoma/leukaemia with prominent nucleoli	Not included
Primary cutaneous MZL	Not included
Transformations of indolent B-cell lymphomas	Not included
Fibrin associated large B-cell lymphoma	Not included
Fluid overload associated B-cell lymphoma	Not included
Primary large-B-cell lymphoma of immune privileged sites	Not included
Hyperplasia in immune deficiency/dysregulation	Not included
Polymorphic lymphoproliferative disorders in immune deficiency/dysregulation	Not included
Lymphomas in immune deficiency/dysregulation	Not included

Follicular Lymphoma

Introduction: FL is a heterogeneous chronic relapsing/remitting B-cell lymphoma, which is both indolent and aggressive with cure in few. Associated with high-grade transformation to DLBCL.

Epidemiology: 5:100,000. Second most common NHL, median age of onset 60, slight male predominance.

Signs/symptoms: Lymphadenopathy and B-symptoms in majority. Marrow involvement common. Rarer include skin or bowel lesions.

FBC: Lymphocytosis and anaemia or thrombocytopenia if marrow involvement. Raised LDH as marker of high-grade transformation.

Blood film: Occasionally lymphocytosis with dense chromatin and deep central clefted nucleus seen.

Diagnosis: Lymph node biopsy. Characteristic t(14;18) on cytogenetics. Germinal cell flow markers. H and E staining showing follicular lymph node involvement. Grade based on centrocyte (small cell)/centroblast (large cell) involvement. Important to differentiate grade 3a (FL) from grade 3b which is treated as DLBCL.

Imaging: PET-CT over contrast CT or MRI.

Lymph node IHC/Flow: Pos: CD10, CD19, CD20, CD22, BCL-2, BCL6. **Variable:** Cyclin D1, CD43, CD45, kappa and lambda light chains. CD21 and CD23 if nodular pattern involving follicular meshwork. **Neg:** CD5, CD30.

Bone marrow biopsy: Useful in grading and therefore tailoring treatment plan in some cases.

Cytogenetics: Characteristic t(14;18) *IgH/BCL2* rearrangement in 85%.

Molecular: *KMT2D, EZH2, CARD11, RB1* and *FOXO1* mutations. Many others associated but these the most common.

Staging: Ann Arbor.

Prognosis: Use of FLIPI at diagnosis for first line treatment. FLIPI2 for PFS based on rituximab treated FL patients.

Other important work up: ECHO, G6PD, virology, immunoglobulins, fertility counselling, LDH.

Tx at diagnosis: Only rarely requires treatment at diagnosis. Majority are under active surveillance unless treatment indication.

Tx indications: Rapidly progressive, organ compression causing symptoms, marrow involvement with cytopaenias, B-symptoms, bulky disease and transformation.

First line tx options: Any stage 3B or above should be treated as DLBCL

Limited stage asymptomatic (1A or 2A non-bulky): Observation, local excision or IFRT if limited.

Advanced stage asymptomatic (3A or above Non-bulky): Observation or single agent rituximab.

<u>Any stage symptomatic</u>: R-CHOP/CVP/bendamustine if FLIPI score 0–1. O-CHOP/CVP/bendamustine if FLIPI score 2–5. Choice of CHOP/CVP/bendamustine based on grading and previous therapy. Consolidation therapy with 2/12 Rituximab or Obinutuzumab for 2 years if PR or CR improves PFS but not OS.

Progression of disease within 2 years (POD24) is a clinically significant endpoint to identify patients with high risk of death.

Second/third line: Observation if asymptomatic. Consider R/O-bendamustine/CVP/CHOP if not used. If responded to first line treatment with good results then repeat. 2 years of Rituximab or Obinutuzumab consolidation again.

Third line or trial options: PI3k inhibitor (can be used second line) vs allograft or trial.

Emergency scenarios: Transformation to DLBCL then treat with R/O-CHOP and consider R/O consolidation for 2 years.

Transplant: Consider auto or allograft in high risk fit patients who respond to second line or R/R disease.

Important side effects of Tx: Reactions to obinutuzumab higher than rituximab.

Supportive care: Antiviral prophylaxis, PPI, antiemetics.

Other considerations: Those who have bendamustine need irradiated products. IFRT of neck patients should have yearly thyroid function.

Trials to quote: <u>PRIMA trial</u>: Rituximab 2-year consolidation improves PFS. <u>GALLIUM trial</u>: Use of Obinutuzumab as first line monoclonal in FL. <u>POD24</u>: Those who relapse within 2 years have inferior outcomes.

Guidelines:

https://rmpartners.nhs.uk/wp-content/uploads/2018/11/PanLondon_FL_Guidelines_Sept2018_v2.pdf

https://b-s-h.org.uk/guidelines/guidelines/guideline-on-the-investigation-and-management-of-follicular-lymphoma/

FLIPI score for overall survival and decision on rituximab or obinutuzumab.

Parameter	Score of 1
Age	> 60
Stage	> 2
LDH	Raised
Hb	< 120 g/L
Sites	> 4

Total score	Risk
0–1	Low
2	Intermediate
3–5	High

FLIPI2 score for estimating PFS in FL.

Parameter	Score of 1
Age	> 60
Bone marrow	Involved
Bet 2 microglobulin	Raised
Hb	< 120 g/L
Biggest node	> 6 cm

Total score	Risk
0–1	Low
2	Intermediate
3–5	High

Mantle Cell Lymphoma

Introduction: Rare mature B-cell lymphoma often presenting with marrow and extranodal disease with indolent and aggressive forms.

Epidemiology: 1:100,000 and 3–10% of all NHL, affects any age but median age 60–70, male predominance of 2–3:1.

Signs/symptoms: Widespread LN, splenomegaly, extranodal involvement in 30–50%, BM involvement, rarely B-symptoms.

FBC/Blood film: Cytopaenias if marrow infiltrated, raised WCC, mantle cells in PB appear as large cells with basophilic cytoplasm, occasional nucleoli and clefted nucleus. In more blastoid morphology chromatin may appear more open with multiple nucleoli.

Diagnosis: Based on LN biopsy morphology, IHC and classical t(11;14). Ki67 impacts grading and survival.

Lymph node IHC/flow: Pos: CD19, 20, 22, 79a, FMC7, BCL2.

Weak/variable: CD5 in most. **Neg:** CD23.

Cytogenetics: In t(11;14) there is an upregulation of Cyclin D1 in 95% of patients due to *BCL1* dysregulation via *IgH* on chromosome 14.

Molecular: Frequently mutated include *ATM*, *CCND1*, *TP53* and *NOTCH1*. *SOX11* mutation often associated with indolent disease.

Staging: Ann Arbor staging.

Tx at diagnosis? Not always. In indolent or asymptomatic disease can monitor. Otherwise divide into transplant eligible or ineligible.

Other important work up: ECHO, G6PD, LDH, B2M, virology, immunoglobulins, HLA typing, PICC, fertility based on treatment.

First line tx options:

Transplant eligible: Nordic protocol with R-MaxiCHOP and R-HDAra-C alternating for 6 cycles or R-DHAP instead of R-HDAra-C. Maintenance rituximab after Autograft for 3 years.

Transplant ineligible: R-CHOP or R-Bendamustine then maintenance Rituximab for 2 years. BTKi if not suitable for high dose chemotherapy. In early-stage disease consider IFRT only first line irrespective of transplant eligibility.

Second/third line: BTKi. Ibrutinib licensed via NHS England. Other BTKi acalabrutinib and zanubrutinib — licensed for use in relapsed disease by FDA but not through NHS England at present. Consider trials and plan for CAR-T or allograft if appropriate.

R-BAC if transplant ineligible other therapies like lenalidomide, bortezomib or venetoclax if able to get funding for compassionate use or enter into a clinical trial.

Prognosis: Depending on morphology and aggressiveness. 8–12-year OS. Use of MIPI and Ki67 give either low, intermediate or high-risk disease corresponding to median survival.

Transplant: Auto in CR/PR1. Allo in CR2, relapse or resistant disease. CAR-T after failure of 2 lines of therapy including BTKi.

Important side effects of tx: Bendamustine: Irradiated blood products.

BTKi: AF, bleeding and hypertension.

Assessing response: Interim PET scan to assess response not recommended but in practice useful.

Supportive care: Antiviral, bacterial and fungal. PCP prophylaxis. Mouthwashes. Eye drops for cytarabine. TLS not common unless bulky disease or high Ki-67.

Trials to quote: LYMA trial: Maintenance rituximab. ZUMA-2: CAR-T in relapsed or refractory mantle cell lymphoma.

Other considerations: CNS prophylaxis if blastoid morphology, high Ki67 or high risk. If GI symptoms, consider OGD to rule out GI disease.

Guidelines:

https://rmpartners.nhs.uk/wp-content/uploads/2020/01/Pan-London-Less-Common-Guidelines-Jan-2020.pdf

https://onlinelibrary.wiley.com/doi/full/10.1111/bjh.15283

MIPI score for prognosis in mantle cell lymphoma.

Score	Age	ECOG performance status	LDH: ULN LDH ratio	WCC ($\times10^9$/L)		Total score	Risk
0	< 50	0–1	< 0.67	< 6.7		0–3	Low
1	50–59	-	0.67–0.99	6.7–9.9		4–6	Intermediate
2	60–69	2–4	1–1.49	10–14.9		6	High
3	≥ 70	-	≥ 1.5	≥ 15			

Diffuse Large B-Cell Lymphoma

Introduction: High-grade aggressive, curable B-cell lymphoma associated with constitutional symptoms and widespread lymphadenopathy.

Epidemiology: Most common lymphoma. 30% of all NHL, increasing incidence with age. Median age 60–70. Slight male predominance.

Signs/symptoms: Lymphadenopathy, B-symptoms (night sweats, weight loss, fever) infections, localised pain, pleural effusions.

FBC/Blood film: Often normal FBC unless marrow involvement which would be in keeping with lymphoma in leukaemic phase

Diagnosis: Biopsy of LN, ideally excision, showing diffuse infiltrate pattern of cells expressing pan-B-cell markers with Ki67 often 80–90%. Germinal centre (GC) and activated B-cell (ABC) subtype based on cell of origin based on immunohistochemistry pattern.

Flow panel/IHC: Pos: CD19, 20, 22, 45 c-MYC, BCL-2 and 6 expression in 20–50% of cases. Cut off value of 40% (MYC) and 50% (BCL-2) for +ve protein expression in IHC. **Weak/variant:** CD10+ in GC. EBV+ **Neg:** CD5, 23,25, TdT.

Cytogenetics/molecular: 30% *BCL2* or *BCL6* translocations. 10% *MYC*. 5–10% double or triple hit translocations.

Staging: Ann Arbor staging via PET. Bulky disease > 7.5 cm.

IPI for prognosis: Age, stage, LDH, PS, extra nodal disease sites.

CNS IPI: IPI + specific extranodal sites involved. Score of 4 or more indicates need for HD-MTX prophylaxis though role remains controversial. Additionally, if > 1 extranodal sites or testes, breast or adrenal involvement for CNS prophylaxis.

Subtypes: GC vs NGC. Double hit vs triple hit. PCNSL, PMBCL, ALK+, T-cell rich DLBCL, de novo vs transformed vs EBV+.

Tx at diagnosis? Yes.

Other important work up: ECHO, G6PD, Virology, immunoglobulins, PICC, fertility counselling based on treatment, LDH.

First line tx options: Early-stage vs advanced stage. R-CHOP standard first line therapy +/- IFRT +/- CNS prophylaxis. R- Polatuzumab-CHP now licensed in first line instead of R-CHOP. R-CHOP below can therefore be interchangeable with R-Polatuzumab-CHP if IPI 2–5.

Stage 1A non-bulky: 4 × R-CHOP and IFRT.

Stage 2A non-bulky: 6 × R-CHOP.

Bulky stage 1/2a: 6 × R-CHOP and IFRT.

Advanced stage: 6 × R-CHOP and IFRT if bulky disease.

Frail: Dose attenuated R-CHOP or R-CVP.

Poor risk or double/triple hit: Consider R-CODOX-M/R-IVAC as first line.

Second line: Relapse within 1 year or refractory: CD19-CAR-T and bridging.

Relapse after 1 year: Salvage chemo i.e. R-ICE and Autograft.

Third line: Clinical trials. R-DHAP, R-ICE or R-CODOX-M/R-IVAC. CAR-T after second line.

Prognosis: Interim PET after 3 cycles to assess Deauville response. End of treatment PET.

5-year OS: 70–80% in low/low-intermediate IPI. 30–40% in high IPI.

Transplant: Autograft in relapsed disease with BEAM or LEAM conditioning. Allo less favourable than CAR-T. Axicabtagene ciloleucel is recommended for adults with DLBCL who have primary refractory disease or who relapse within one year of treatment or in third line patients.

Important side effects of tx: Anthracycline toxicity, peripheral neuropathy, rituximab reactions, CRS and ICANS in CAR-T.

Trials to quote: ZUMA-1: CAR-T in relapsed refractory DLBCL. ZUMA-7: Randomised trial of CAR-T versus auto in patients who have primary refractory disease or who relapse within 1 year of first line therapy. POLARIX: R-Pola-CHP improves PFS and OS in IPI > 1.

Supportive care: TLS prophylaxis in bulky disease with rasburicase. Antiviral, fungal and bacterial prophylaxis.

Other considerations: CNS prophylaxis as above. CAR-T consideration if relapsed or refractory following 1st or 2nd line.

Guidelines:

https://rmpartners.nhs.uk/wp-content/uploads/2020/01/Pan-London-DLBCL-Guidelines-Jan-2020.pdf

https://www.nice.org.uk/guidance/NG52/chapter/Recommendations#management-of-diffuse-large-bcell-lymphoma

IPI in DLBCL for OS risk stratification.

Parameter	Score of 1
Age	> 60
Stage	> 2
LDH	> 1 × ULN
ECOG Performance status	> 1
Extranodal sites	> 1

Total score	Risk
0–1	Low
2	Intermediate
> 2	High

CNS-IPI score for assessing risk of CNS disease progression/relapse in DLBCL.

Parameter	Score of 1
Age	> 60
ECOG performance status	> 1
LDH	Raised
Stage	> 1
Extranodal sites	> 1
Kidney or adrenal involvement?	Yes

Total score	Risk
0–1	Low
2–3	Intermediate
> 3	High

Primary CNS Lymphoma

Introduction: High-grade lymphoma, predominantly DLBCL, in the CNS with no other site. Rarer forms include T-cell or Burkitt's.

Epidemiology: 1% of NHL, 90% are DLBCL in origin. < 1:100,000 incidence. 65–70 median age of onset. No sex predominance.

Signs/symptoms: B-symptoms, headache, visual disturbances, seizures, other focal neurology.

Diagnosis: Biopsy or CSF proven flow markers/IHC with PET-CT showing no nodal disease. 10–20% intraocular involvement.

Flow panel/IHC: Pos: B-cell markers, CD45, BCL2 and 6, MUM1, IRF4, MYC. **Neg:** TdT, CD10, 30, 38, 138.

Cytogenetics/molecular: *MYD88* and *BCL6* rearrangements/mutations seen.

Staging: MRI of head with contrast as well as PET to assess avidity and rule out systemic disease.

Tx at diagnosis? Yes.

Other important work up: ECHO, G6PD, virology, immunoglobulins and paraprotein, PICC, fertility counselling, LP if biopsy tough, creatinine clearance and testicular USS if under 60 years old, LDH.

First line tx options:

Induction: High dose MTX regime such as MATRIX for 4 cycles if fit and PS < 3 followed by interim PET after 2 cycles and EOTPET.

Consolidation: Autograft.

Frail patients:

Induction: Rituximab, MTX, procarbazine and temozolomide. Consider best supportive care also.

Maintenance: Oral procarbazine or whole brain radiotherapy.

Second/third line: Clinical trial, R-ICE, autograft or consider CAR-T/allograft if multiple relapsed/refractory disease.

Prognosis: 2-year OS-60–70%. Poor OS (3–4 months) in relapsed/refractory disease.

Transplant: Yes, auto consolidation in CR/PR or SD with good PS. Allo not common unless refractory disease and suitable patient.

Important side effects of tx: MTX toxicity and ensure creatinine clearance > 45 ml/min before starting.

Trials to quote: IELSG32: Addition of rituximab and thiotepa to HD MTX and cytarabine improves 2 year-OS.

Supportive care: Antiviral, fungal and bacterial. No septrin for PCP prophylaxis due to MTX interaction. Mouthwashes. Eye drops.

Other considerations: Avoid steroids pre-biopsy. HIV testing as can be HIV associated. MRI to diagnose if biopsy not possible.

Guidelines: https://onlinelibrary.wiley.com/doi/full/10.1111/bjh.15661?af=R
https://www.pathologyoutlines.com/topic/lymphomaprimaryCNSlymphoma.html

Primary Mediastinal B-Cell Lymphoma

Introduction: High-grade B-cell lymphoma of thymic origin presenting as bulky mediastinal mass commonly expressing CD30.

Epidemiology: 2–4% of all NHL, predominantly in young adults, median age 30–35-years-old. Slight female predominance of 1.2:1.

Signs/symptoms: Fever, weight loss, night sweats, chest pain, palpitations. Compressive symptoms include SOB and symptoms of SVCO.

Diagnosis: LN biopsy of mass showing thymic origin B-cells distinct from DLBCL, either GC or ABC can be CD30+.

Flow panel/IHC: Pos: CD19, 20, 22, 79b. **Variable:** CD30+. **Neg:** EBV, CD5, sIgM, CD15.

Cytogenetics/molecular: 9q amplification of genes CD274 and *PDCDILG2*. Dysregulation of JAK-STAT and NFkB pathways.

Staging: PET-CT scan. Ann Arbor staging. End of treatment PET-CT recommended. IPI often low due to age so use age adjusted.

Tx at diagnosis? Yes.

Other important work up: ECHO, G6PD, virology, PICC, fertility counselling based on treatment, LDH.

First line tx options: 6 × R-CHOP14 with GCSF support and IFRT. DA-EPOCH-R without IFRT is another option if IFRT contraindicated or not suitable. Consider omission of IFRT if end of treatment PET-CT -ve in DA-EPOCH-R.

Second/third line: Clinical trial. Same salvage as DLBCL i.e., R-ICE, R-DHAP. IFRT if not given before in localised relapse. Consideration of other agents such as brentuximab or CAR-T.

Prognosis: 5-year OS 80–95% in R-CHOP or DA-EPOCH-R.

Transplant: Autograft consolidation in relapsed/refractory disease.

Important side effects of tx: As for R-CHOP mentioned above. DA-EPOCH-R need bloods during first cycle to calculate dose adjustment.

Trials to quote: UK NCRI R-CHOP 14 vs 21 trial: Better outcomes in 14-day vs 21-day cycle.

Supportive care: As for R-CHOP mentioned above. Cardiac monitoring if ECG changes prior to treatment and cardiology review.

Other considerations: CNS prophylaxis calculated as per other lymphomas. If SVCO give high dose steroids and urgent radiotherapy.

Guidelines:
https://onlinelibrary.wiley.com/doi/full/10.1111/bjh.15731
https://ashpublications.org/blood/article/132/8/782/39454/How-I-treat-primary-mediastinal-B-cell-lymphoma

Marginal Zone Lymphoma

Introduction: Indolent lymphoma with 3 subtypes arising from post-germinal centre B-cells in the marginal zone.

Epidemiology: 11% of all NHL, relatively rare. Associated with atypical infections, Sjogren's syndrome in MALT lymphoma of salivary gland and Hashimoto's thyroiditis in thyroid MALT lymphoma. Median age of 50, 60 and 70 in nodal, extranodal and SMZL respectively.

Signs/symptoms: B symptoms, lymphadenopathy in nodal type, splenomegaly in SMZL, GI symptoms, symptoms at disease site, autoimmune complications in SMZL and paraprotein.

FBC/Blood film: Lymphocytosis with cytoplasmic villous projections from lymphocytes, anaemia or thrombocytopaenia due to hypersplenism. Typically, no lymphocytosis or film changes in other forms.

Diagnosis: LN or site of disease biopsy with characteristic flow pattern +/- morphology +/- viral infection in MALT.

Lymph node IHC:

MZL: **Pos:** CD19, FMC7. **Weak/variable:** CD103, MALT (50%) BCL10+. **Neg:** CD5, 11c, 23, 25, BCL-2.

SMZL: **Pos:** CD19 ,20, 79b, SmIg (IgM > IgG, IgD), FMC7 and kappa light chain restricted. **Weak/variable:** Most are CD23+.

Neg: CD5, 10, 11c, 25, 103.

Bone marrow: As above for flow and morphology. Useful in staging of disease. Diffuse nodular lymphoid infiltrate.

Cytogenetics:

MALT: t(11;18) and t(1;14) poor response to *H. Pylori* eradication in gastric.

SMZL: 7q deletion. 80% of all subtypes have cytogenetic abnormalities and highly varied.

Staging: TNM in gastric MALT. Others are staged by Ann Arbor.

Subtypes: Extranodal (gastric and non-gastric), nodal and splenic.

Tx at diagnosis? Gastric MALT: Yes if *H. Pylori* positive. All subtypes no if asymptomatic. Indications to treat: GI bleeding, bulky disease, cytopaenia or symptoms are reason to initiate treatment otherwise close monitoring.

Other important work up: ECHO, G6PD, LDH, B2M, DAT, virology, immunoglobulins and paraprotein, serology for chlamydia, campylobacter, HCV and *Borrelia burgdorferi*, *H. Pylori*, fertility counselling based on treatment.

First line tx options:

SMZL: Single agent rituximab or combination with CVP or R-Benda. HCV related Peg-IFN and ribavirin.

Nodal disease: Stage1 disease: IFRT. Stage 2: IFRT + rituximab-based chemotherapy as per FL regimes R-CVP.

Extranodal: *Gastric MALT stage 1/2 disease*: H pylori eradication with triple therapy of 2 antibiotics and PPI.

Non-gastric MALT: IFRT for localised disease, rituximab monotherapy or in combination, doxycycline for ocular disease.

Second/third line:

SMZL: Splenic irradiation, splenectomy, R-CHOP if resistant/aggressive disease. Clinical trial. Consider CAR-T, BTKi or lenalidomide.

Nodal disease: R-CHOP or regime not tried in first line. Clinical trial.

Extranodal: R-CHOP, R-CVP or other systemic therapy. If asymptomatic with residual disease yearly OGD.

Prognosis:

Gastric MALT: 5-year OS 80–90%.

SMZL: Median OS > 10 years with 10% never needing treatment. Poor prognostic signs include: High LDH, TP53 mutation, cytopaenias, high white cell count, low albumin. Chromosome 7 abnormalities.

Nodal: Median OS > 10 years.

Transplant: Rarely considered unless resistant or high-grade transformations.

Assessing response: Follow up OGD 6, 12 and 24 months in gastric MALT. Other forms would usually do an end of treatment scan.

Supportive care: Antiviral prophylaxis. No need for others unless severe infection or neutropaenia.

Other considerations: Irradiated products if using fludarabine. Pneumovax is splenic irradiation/splenectomy.

Guidelines:

https://rmpartners.nhs.uk/wp-content/uploads/2020/01/Pan-London-Less-Common-Guidelines-Jan-2020.pdf

https://bhs.be/storage/app/media/userfiles/files/Guidelines/Marginal_Zone_Lymphomas_2014.pdf

Burkitt's Lymphoma

Introduction: Rare high-grade, aggressive but curable B-cell lymphoma which if untreated is life threatening.

Epidemiology: 2.5:1,000,000 per year. Endemic Burkitt's in childhood seen in Africa associated with EBV infection. Median age 31. Male sex predominance of 2.5:1.

Signs/symptoms: Widespread large LN, often intra-abdominal, B symptoms, weight loss, extranodal tumours in EBV associated version often affecting bones such as mandible. Marrow involvement leading to cytopaenias, CNS disease.

FBC/Blood film: Cytopaenias and circulating Burkitt cells may be seen.

Diagnosis: LN biopsy showing Ki67 of close to 100%, BM morphology.

Flow pane/LN IHC: Pos: CD10, 19, 20, 22, BCL-6, Smlg. **Neg:** CD5, 23 and TdT. Ki67 in DLBCL < 90%, in Burkitt's > 99%.

Bone marrow/LN: "Starry sky" appearance of large B-lymphoblasts with multiple nucleoli, open chromatin, and thin rim of cytoplasm.

Cytogenetics/molecular: t(8;14) in 80%, t(2;8) in 15–20%. t(14;18) poor prognostic sign.

Staging: Ann Arbor staging with CT and PET-CT. Poor prognostic risk factors include > 40-years-old, advanced stage, CNS disease, high LDH, no CR after 2 cycles or poor ECOG performance status.

Tx at diagnosis? YES! Urgent treatment with TLS prophylaxis with rasburicase.

Other important work up: ECHO, G6PD, virology, LDH, immunoglobulins, creatinine clearance, PICC, fertility counselling based on treatment, MRI or LP.

First line tx options:

Low risk or > 60: 3 × R-CODOX-M for 3 cycles.

High risk or < 60: R-CODOX-M/R-IVAC × 2 cycles each. 4 in total.

DA-EPOCH-R or R-CHOP in those not able to tolerate most intense regimes.

Second/third line: R-ICE or other salvage chemotherapy regimens with autograft consolidation.

Prognosis: CR in 60–80% of high risk and in 90% of low-risk patients. Follow up until > 2 years post treatment. Relapses usually occur in first year.

Transplant: Autograft in those who do not achieve CR or who relapse. Allograft rarely performed.

Important side effects of tx: TLS, mucositis, MTX toxicity, above-mentioned side effects of other chemotherapy.

Supportive care: TLS prophylaxis, mouthwashes for mucositis, antiviral, antibacterial, antifungal and PCP prophylaxis, eye drops for cytarabine, IV hydration for MTX.

Other considerations: 30% associated with EBV. Associated HIV infection may be present and should be treated with antiretroviral therapy in combination with SACT in specialist HIV centre. Most Burkitt's managed in tertiary centre if high risk.
IT MTX if no other CNS penetrating agents given in chemotherapy.
Guidelines:
https://rmpartners.nhs.uk/wp-content/uploads/2020/01/Pan-London-Less-Common-Guidelines-Jan-2020.pdf

Waldenström's Macroglobulinaemia

Introduction: Rare B-cell lymphoma with associated IgM paraprotein, clonal LPL cells and commonly *MYD88* mutated.

Epidemiology: Increased risk of developing WM in autoimmune disorders such as Sjogren's or SLE. Risk of WM from IgM MGUS 1–2% per year. Disease of the elderly. Commonly > 65. Male predominance.

Signs/symptoms: Splenomegaly, anaemia, lymph nodes, symptoms of hyperviscosity such as SOB, cytopaenias and disease burden symptoms.

FBC/Blood film: LPL cells seen as small to medium lymphocytes with basophilic cytoplasm and eccentric nucleus.

Diagnosis:

IgM MGUS:

- IgM Paraprotein < 30 g/L.
- Asymptomatic.
- BM clear of LPL infiltrate.

WM/LPL:

- Paraprotein > 30 g/l.
- BM or LN LPL cell involvement.
- Clinical symptoms +/- *MYD88* mutation.

Lymph node IHC/flow: Pos: Pan B-cell markers as well as surface IgM, CD38+. **Neg:** CD5 and 10.

Bone marrow: Infiltration of clonal population mentioned above. Recommended to do at diagnosis.

Cytogenetics/molecular: *MYD88* mutation most common. *CXCR4* mutation in 40%. *TP53* mutation in 10%, associated with a worse OS.

Staging: Ann Arbor, CT staging recommended as minimum, PET-CT not recommended but often done in diagnostic work up.

Tx at diagnosis? No, if asymptomatic monitor. Risk of progression to symptoms is 60% at 5 years.

Indications for treatment: B symptoms, splenomegaly, cytopaenias, bulky LN, IgM or paraprotein related phenomena.

Other important work up: ECHO, G6PD, LDH, B2M, virology, immunoglobulins and paraprotein, SFLC, Cryoglobulins, cold agglutinins, ophthalmology review if signs of hyperviscosity. VWD screen, anti-MAG antibodies.

Emergency scenarios:

Hyperviscosity: Seen when IgM > 40 g/L. IVF and plasmapheresis. Refer to tertiary centre generally. Refer to ophthalmology to assess.

Acquired VWD: Rare complication. Treat with IVIG, plasmapheresis and VWF concentrates. Refer to tertiary coagulation specialist centre!

First line tx options:
Chemo: Bortezomib or dexamethasone in combination with cyclophosphamide and rituximab. R-benda also used.

BTKi: Ibrutinib or Zanubrutinib NICE approved after first line and better in *MYD88* mutated. Single agent rituximab in more frail patients.

Second/third line: Different BTKi, rituximab, bortezomib regime, autograft if less than PR or clinical trials.

Prognosis: 5-year OS in low, intermediate and high risk: 85%, 65%, 35% respectively.

ISSWM: Age, haemoglobin, platelets, B2M and paraprotein concentration to stratify risk but not guide treatment decisions.

Transplant: Autograft as above. Allograft in high-risk disease which have failed 2 lines including BTKi.

Important side effects of tx: IgM flare after rituximab initiation. Avoid transfusion until IgM reduced if possible.

Response:
CR: Absence of IgM and normal BM. Resolution of LN or splenomegaly.

VGPR: 90% reduction in IgM from baseline + criteria above.

PR: > 50% reduction but < 90% in IgM. Reduction in LN or splenomegaly. No new symptoms.

Minor response: > 25% reduction but < 50% in IgM. No new symptoms.

Stable disease: < 25% reduction or < 25% increase in IgM.

Progressive disease: > 25% increase in IgM and/or new symptoms.

Supportive care: Antiviral and PCP prophylaxis, hypogammaglobulinemia consider antibacterial prophylaxis. Pneumovax for all patients. Irradiated blood products if exposed to Bendamustine.

Other considerations: IgM associated neuropathy. Exclude CNS disease. High-grade transformation can occur. Bing-Neel syndrome or AL Amyloidosis can occur and are indications for treatment.

Guidelines:
https://onlinelibrary.wiley.com/doi/full/10.1111/bjh.18036

T-Cell Lymphomas

Peripheral T-Cell Lymphoma NOS

Introduction: Rare and aggressive nodal T-cell lymphoma with some extranodal features seen. Diagnosed when no other WHO T-cell lymphoma subtype criteria are met based on histology, flow and molecular. Heterogenous group of conditions.

Epidemiology: 4% of all lymphomas and half of all T-cell lymphomas. Can affect any age but median age 62 years. Slight male predominance.

Signs/symptoms: Lymphadenopathy, splenomegaly, constitutional symptoms, pleural effusions, occasionally rashes.

Diagnosis: LN biopsy or bone marrow biopsy with characteristic flow panel.

Flow panel/IHC: Pos: CD4, 8 with TCR rearrangement and clonality. **Neg:** Varies but aberrant CD5 and 7 expression.

Cytogenetics/molecular: Loss of 5q, 9q, 12q in 30%. Share gene expression profile with AITL in 20%. TCR rearrangements.

Staging: Ann Arbor by CT, consider marrow and PET-CT for extranodal disease sites, IPI and CNS-IPI useful though not so helpful in other extranodal T-cell lymphomas.

Tx at diagnosis? Yes, often presenting as late stage.

Other important work up: ECHO, G6PD, virology, immunoglobulins, HLA typing, PICC, fertility counselling based on treatment, LDH.

First line tx options: Always consider trial due to aggressive nature. 6 cycles of CHOP +/- etoposide. Radiotherapy if bulky disease.

Second/third line: CHOEP, GEM-P, ICE with allograft. Brentuximab if CD30+. Consider bendamustine, purine analogous, alemtuzumab, pralatrexate and romidepsin as trial agents if available.

Prognosis: Poor prognosis in all stages but worse in later. 5-year OS for all 30%. Relapse after CR1 common during first 2 years.

Transplant: Auto in CR1 and consider allo in relapse or young and fit with matched donor.

Important side effects of tx: Irradiated blood products in purine analogues and bendamustine.

Supportive care: Antibacterial, viral and fungal prophylaxis. Consider PCP prophylaxis as per regime.

Trials to quote for all T-cell lymphomas: International T-cell lymphoma project (ITLP) for all T-cell lymphomas.

Guidelines:
https://b-s-h.org.uk/media/2895/t-nhl-guideline-3-8-13-updated-with-changes-accepted-v1-rg.pdf

Angioimmunoblastic T-Cell Lymphoma

Introduction: Aggressive rare peripheral T-cell lymphoma, with immune phenomena seen and B and T-cell clones present.

Epidemiology: 20% of peripheral T-cell lymphomas. Incidence 1:1,000,000 in the UK. 2% of all NHL. Commonly in older adults. Median age 62. No sex predominance. Often a delay in diagnosis.

Signs/symptoms: Lymphadenopathy, hepatosplenomegaly, rash, constitutional symptoms, eosinophilia, HLH and autoimmune complications such as AIHA or cold agglutinins present, hypergammaglobulinemia, raised LDH.

Diagnosis: Tough to diagnose. IHC from LN showing malignant T-cells with background of B-cell rich populations and TCR gene clonality via Rt-PCR with characteristic flow panel below. Loss of LN follicular network and neovascularisation.

Flow panel/IHC: Pos: CD4, 10, 21 if follicular cells present, BCL6, CXCL13, CXCR3. **Neg:** Reduced CD8 expression compared to CD4.CD3 and CD7 can also be negative.

Cytogenetics/molecular: Additional X chromosome, trisomy 5. *IDH2*, *TET2* and *IRF4* mutations.

Staging: Ann Arbor by CT, consider marrow and PET-CT for extranodal disease sites.

Tx at diagnosis? Yes, often presenting as late stage but treat any stage.

Other important work up: ECHO, G6PD, virology, immunoglobulins, HLA typing, PICC, fertility counselling based on treatment, HTLV-1, LDH.

First line tx options: Always consider trial due to aggressive nature. CHOP, CVP or CHOEP. Fludarabine/cyclophosphamide also used.

Second/third line: Immunomodulatory agents such as lenalidomide combined with steroids. Ciclosporin. Brentuximab if CD30+.

Prognosis: 3-year OS 60% if CR1 and auto. 5-year OS 33% in patients from ITLP.

Transplant: Auto in CR1 or in relapse. Allograft if donor, suitable recipient and high risk or relapsed disease.

Important side effects of tx: Irradiated products in fludarabine. Managing autoimmune phenomena.

Supportive care: Antibacterial, viral and fungal prophylaxis. Consider PCP prophylaxis as per regime.

Guidelines:
https://b-s-h.org.uk/media/2895/t-nhl-guideline-3-8-13-updated-with-changes-accepted-v1-rg.pdf

Anaplastic Large Cell Lymphoma

Introduction: Rare lymphoma with 3 distinct subtypes of cutaneous form, and ALK+/-nodal forms which often present late.

Epidemiology: 3–5% of NHL. Rare variant associated with breast implants also. 1 in 100,000. ALK+ slight male predominance.

ALK+: Median age 30. ALK-: Median age 45–60.

Signs/symptoms: B symptoms, bulky LN, extranodal involvement i.e., skin and liver.

Diagnosis: LN biopsy with TCR gene rearrangements, clonal population of large lymphocytes, ALK status. CD30+ in 60%.

Flow panel/IHC: Pos: As above and EMA, TCR gene rearrangements. **Variants:** CD30+ in ALK+. **Neg:** CD3, EBV.

Cytogenetics/molecular: t(2;5) *NPM1:ALK*.

Staging: Ann Arbor staging with CT. IPI has its use, but ALK status is best indicator. CNS involvement rare.

Tx at diagnosis? Yes.

Other important work up: ECHO, G6PD, virology, immunoglobulins, HLA typing, PICC, fertility counselling based on treatment, LDH.

First line tx options: Always consider trial.

Limited stage: 4 × CHOP and IFRT.

Advanced: 6–8 × CHOP. Brentuximab if CD30+. Local excision for cutaneous forms with IFRT.

ALK-: Treat as PTCL NOS.

Second/third line: Brentuximab if not used before. Platinum based regime. Trial. Auto consolidation or allo if appropriate.

Prognosis:

ALK+: better prognosis than ALK- with 5-year OS 70% and 55% respectively.

Cutaneous: 10-year OS 90–95%.

Transplant: In relapse or CR1 in high-risk disease.

Supportive care: Antibacterial, viral and fungal prophylaxis. Consider PCP as per regime.

Guidelines:

https://b-s-h.org.uk/media/2895/t-nhl-guideline-3-8-13-updated-with-changes-accepted-v1-rg.pdf

Mycosis Fungoides (MFU)/Sezary Syndrome (SS)

Introduction: The most common cutaneous T-cell lymphoma which in leukaemic form is known as SS.

Epidemiology: Rare NHL though represents 50% of cutaneous T-cell lymphomas. Median age of onset 55–60, 2:1 male predominance.

Signs/symptoms: SS: Erythroderma, lymphadenopathy and cerebriform clonal lymphocytes. MFU: Skin lesions and LN.

Diagnosis: Based on morphology, IHC, cerebriform nucleus in lymphoid infiltrate in epidermis with Langerhans cells.

Flow panel/IHC: Pos: CD2, 3, 4, 45RO and 8, TCR beta gene rearrangement. **Variant:** CD30. **Neg:** CD7 and 26.

Staging: TNMB staging system. T = % of skin involvement. N = nodes involved. M = visceral involvement. B = circulating cells in PB.

Tx at diagnosis? Yes.

Other important work up: ECHO, G6PD, virology, immunoglobulins, HLA typing, PICC, fertility counselling based on treatment, HTLV-1, LDH.

First line tx options:

Early stage (1–2): SDT, phototherapy or radiotherapy.

2B: SDT, Bexarotene or IFN.

Late stage 3–4: MTX, ECP, trials.

Second/third line: Always consider trial.

Early stage (1–2): 2B first line options. 2B: Brentuximab, mogamulizumab.

Late stage 3–4: Brentuximab, mogamulizumab or alemtuzumab. Chemotherapy in all stages as third line treatment.

Prognosis: Worse prognosis in late-stage disease or in transformed large T-cell lymphoma.

Transplant: In relapse or CR1 where appropriate.

Trials to quote: MAVORIC: Mogamulizumab use in refractory or relapsed disease.

Supportive care: Antibacterial, viral and fungal prophylaxis. Consider PCP prophylaxis as per regime. Managing pruritis.

Guidelines:

https://b-s-h.org.uk/media/2895/t-nhl-guideline-3-8-13-updated-with-changes-accepted-v1-rg.pdf

https://rmpartners.nhs.uk/wp-content/uploads/2020/01/Pan-London-Less-Common-Guidelines-Jan-2020.pdf

NK-Cell Lymphoma

Introduction: Extranodal very rare T-cell lymphoma associated with EBV and with nasal involvement. Chronic LPD of NK-cells and aggressive NK leukaemia not covered here.

Epidemiology: More common in Asian populations though still rare. Median age of 50–60 with male predominance of 3:1.

Signs/symptoms: Depends on site of disease. Can involve sinuses, gut, testes or BM as well as other extranodal sites. Occasionally LN disease.

Diagnosis: Based on clonality, flow panel, extranodal involvement, commonly nasal/sinuses and EBV+.

Flow panel/IHC: Pos: CD2, 56, 3ε EBV. **Neg:** No TCR gene rearrangement.

Staging: Ann Arbor. PET-CT for extranodal disease. IPI not useful. CNS involvement uncommon. MRI head to assess nasal cavity.

Tx at diagnosis? Yes.

Other important work up: ECHO, G6PD, virology, immunoglobulins, HLA typing, PICC, fertility counselling based on treatment, ENT review, LDH.

First line tx options:

Localised disease: Asparaginase based regime such as LVDP or DeVIC with IFRT.

Advanced stage: Intensive asparaginase regime such as SMILE or P-GEMOX.

Second/third line: Clinical trial. More aggressive regime than at diagnosis if not used and transplant. Consider pembrolizumab or other checkpoint inhibitors if able to access. Brentuximab if CD30+.

Prognosis: Very poor with late diagnosis common. 5-year OS 20–35%.

Transplant: Not recommended but if appropriate donor or relapse most would consider.

Supportive care: Antibacterial, viral and fungal prophylaxis. Consider PCP as per regime.

Guidelines:

https://b-s-h.org.uk/media/2895/t-nhl-guideline-3-8-13-updated-with-changes-accepted-v1-rg.pdf

https://rmpartners.nhs.uk/wp-content/uploads/2020/01/Pan-London-Less-Common-Guidelines-Jan-2020.pdf

Enteropathy Associated T-Cell Lymphoma

Introduction: Rare, aggressive lymphoma of mature T-cells affecting bowel and associated with HLA DQ2 and 8 and Coeliac disease.

Epidemiology: More common in Europe or Coeliac endemic regions. 1:1,000,000 diagnoses in UK. Adult onset often with undiagnosed Coeliac disease, median age 55. Slight male predominance.

Signs/symptoms: Abdominal pain, diarrhoea, weight loss, GI bleeding, splenomegaly, dermatitis herpetiformis.

Diagnosis: Large T-cells on biopsy, commonly involves jejunum and ileum. 2 subtypes based chromosomal analysis.

Flow panel/IHC: Pos: CD8, 56, 3e, TIA-1. **Neg:** EBV-, CD4, 5.

Cytogenetics/molecular:

EATL type 1: +9q or -16q, associated with HLA DQ2.

EATL type 2: +1q, 5q, 8q.

Staging: Difficult to stage but GI biopsy, CT and BMAT as minimum. IPI of no use.

Tx at diagnosis? Yes.

Other important work up: ECHO, G6PD, virology, immunoglobulins, HLA typing, PICC, fertility counselling based on treatment.

First line tx options: Consider trial at outset. CHOP based therapy with auto consolidation.

Second/third line: Clinical trial. Intercalated CHOP with IVE and HD MTX.

Prognosis: Very poor OS of less than a year. 5-year OS 20%. Rarity may skew statistics.

Transplant: Auto consolidation in CR1 or relapse. Allo in high-risk disease or relapse.

Supportive care: Antibacterial, viral and fungal prophylaxis. Consider PCP as per regime. Nutritional plan.

Guidelines:

https://b-s-h.org.uk/media/2895/t-nhl-guideline-3-8-13-updated-with-changes-accepted-v1-rg.pdf

https://rmpartners.nhs.uk/wp-content/uploads/2020/01/Pan-London-Less-Common-Guidelines-Jan-2020.pdf

https://ashpublications.org/blood/article/118/1/148/28418/Enteropathy-associated-T-cell-lymphoma-clinical

Hepatosplenic T-Cell Lymphoma

Introduction: Rare, aggressive lymphoma of T-cells associated with chronic inflammatory states or immunosuppression.

Epidemiology: Very rare. Seen post-transplant. < 1% of all NHL. Male predominance. Median age of onset 30–35.

Signs/symptoms: Constitutional symptoms, involvement of skin, liver, spleen, marrow. LN rare. B symptoms. Risk of secondary HLH.

Diagnosis: Sinusoidal infiltration of clonal cells with below mentioned phenotype.

Flow panel/IHC: Pos: CD2, 3, 7, 45, 56 and TIA-1. **Neg:** CD4, 5, 8, EBV-.

Cytogenetics/molecular: Gamma-delta T-cell receptor expression and isochrome 7q. Alpha-beta T-cell receptor variant also seen as well as activating mutations of the JAK/STAT pathway.

Staging: Often stage 4 at diagnosis. Biopsy crucial.

Tx at diagnosis? Yes.

Other important work up: ECHO, G6PD, virology, immunoglobulins, HLA typing, PICC, fertility counselling based on treatment, LDH.

First line tx options: Clinical trial. CHOP or alemtuzumab and purine analogue.

Second/third line: Clinical trial. Allo if not done in CR1 before.

Prognosis: Rarely survivors. Too rare to give accurate OS.

Transplant: Allo in CR1.

Supportive care: Antibacterial, viral and fungal prophylaxis. Consider PCP as per regime. Irradiated products if PA.

Guidelines:

https://b-s-h.org.uk/media/2895/t-nhl-guideline-3-8-13-updated-with-changes-accepted-v1-rg.pdf

https://rmpartners.nhs.uk/wp-content/uploads/2020/01/Pan-London-Less-Common-Guidelines-Jan-2020.pdf

https://ashpublications.org/blood/article/136/18/2018/461707/Hepatosplenic-T-cell-lymphoma-a-rare-but

Subcutaneous Panniculitis T-Cell Lymphoma

Introduction: Rarest T-cell lymphoma associated with skin nodules and indolent and aggressive forms.

Epidemiology: 1% of T-cell lymphomas affecting any age. Male predominance. Median age 35-years-old.

Signs/symptoms: Multiple indurated skin nodules, B symptoms, HLH, cytopaenias.

Diagnosis: Biopsy of nodule with clonal gamma-delta or alpha-beta T-cells.

Flow panel/IHC: Pos: CD3 and CD8. Can be CD8+/CD56- or CD8-/CD56+. **Neg:** CD4, 30 and EBV.

Staging: No universal system but BM or other organ involvement is advanced stage.

Tx at diagnosis? Yes.

Other important work up: ECHO, G6PD, virology, immunoglobulins, HLA typing, PICC, fertility counselling based on treatment, LDH.

First line tx options:

Localised disease: IFRT and steroids.

Advanced: CHOP.

Second/third line: Clinical trial. Dose intensified CHOP or IVE /ICE with autograft consolidation but varied consensus.

Prognosis: Variable based on subtype and if HLH present. Worse if HLH and gamma-delta compared to alpha-beta and no HLH.

Transplant: Auto in relapse or CR1 with advanced stage. Consider allo in relapse.

Supportive care: Antibacterial, viral and fungal prophylaxis. Consider PCP as per regime.

Guidelines:

https://b-s-h.org.uk/media/2895/t-nhl-guideline-3-8-13-updated-with-changes-accepted-v1-rg.pdf

https://rmpartners.nhs.uk/wp-content/uploads/2020/01/Pan-London-Less-Common-Guidelines-Jan-2020.pdf

https://ashpublications.org/blood/article/111/2/838/103709/Subcutaneous-panniculitis-like-T-cell-lymphoma

Hodgkin Lymphoma

Introduction: CD30+ lymphoma with 2 distinct forms of classical disease (cHL) and NLPHL.

Epidemiology: 15% of all lymphomas. NLPHL rare accounting for 5% of all Hodgkin Lymphoma. Bimodal peak of TYA and middle-aged adults. Slight male predominance.

Signs/symptoms: B-symptoms, lymphadenopathy, and immune symptoms commonly.

Diagnosis: LN biopsy with pathognomonic CD30+ Reed Sternberg cells in cHL or popcorn cells expressing CD20 in NLPHL.

Flow panel/IHC: Pos: CD15, 30, PAX5, PD-L1. **Variable:** EBV+, CD20 in NLPHL. **Neg:** CD2, 3, 10, 45.

Cytogenetics/molecular: Multiple molecular mutations including *BTK*, *CARD11* and *BCL10*.

Staging: PET-CT scan. Ann Arbor staging. BMAT not recommended. Unfavourable prognosis for early stage based on GHSG and EORTC criteria. Presence of 1 or more of the criteria is enough to deem as unfavourable risk. Hasenclever IPS score in advance stage for prognostication.

Tx at diagnosis? Yes.

Other important work up: ECHO, G6PD, virology, PICC, fertility counselling based on treatment, immunoglobulins, ESR, lung function, LDH.

First line tx options: ABVD treatment of choice but other options such as BEACOPP can be justified in certain disease phenotypes.

Early stage favourable: ABVD × 2 → iPET → CMR → AVD × 2 or IFRT or AVD × 1 and IFRT → EOTPET.

OR ABVD × 2 → iPET → PR → Escalated BEACOPP × 2 and IFRT → EOTPET.

Early stage unfavourable: ABVD × 2 → iPET → CMR → AVD × 2 and IFRT or AVD × 4 → EOTPET.

OR ABVD × 2 → iPET → PR → Escalated BEACOPP × 2 and IFRT → EOTPET.

You can start with escalated BEACOPP at first line with 2 cycles then 2 ABVD before PET though not usually done in the UK.

Advanced stage: ABVD × 2 → iPET → CMR → AVD → EOTPET.

OR Escalated BEACOPP × 2 → iPET → CMR → escalated BEACOPP × 2 or AVD × 4 → EOTPET.

If in PR not CR: ABVD × 2 → iPET → PR → Escalated BEACOPP → EOTPET → +/- IFRT.

OR Escalated BEACOPP × 2 → iPET → PR → Escalated BEACOPP × 4 → EOTPET → +/- IFRT.

NLPHL early stage: Surgical excision and IFRT.

NLPHL late stage: R-CVP, R-ABVD or R-CHOP.

Second/third line: Salvage therapy with platinum regime such as ESHAP, DHAP or ICE with consolidation auto if CR.

<u>Fail to respond to salvage therapy</u>: Brentuximab monotherapy or combination therapy such as bendamustine. Brentuximab licensed after autograft and 2 lines of therapy. Consider checkpoint inhibitors such as nivolumab or pembrolizumab though not NICE approved and likely only accessible through trial or compassionate use. Clinical trial.

Prognosis: 80% cured with first line treatment. OS varies based on stage and IPS but most patients OS 75–90%.

Transplant: Autograft in relapsed disease with CR to salvage. Allo in relapsed disease without CR to salvage or relapse after auto.

Important side effects of tx: Lung toxicity with bleomycin. Photosensitive rash. Severe nausea. Cardiotoxicity.

Trials to quote: <u>RATHL</u>: Use of iPET to tailor treatment decisions and drop bleomycin if the iPET negative to reduce lung toxicity risk.

Supportive care: Antiviral and PCP prophylaxis. Steroids for bleomycin and dacarbazine toxicity. Allopurinol. Antiemetics.

Other considerations: Breast cancer screening and thyroid function for those who have had IFRT to head and neck. MDS monitoring and other cancers. Lung function monitoring for signs or symptoms. Irradiated products for life.

Guidelines:
https://www.kingshealthpartners.org/assets/000/003/344/Pan_London_Hodgkin_Guidelines_Jan_2020_original.pdf
https://onlinelibrary.wiley.com/doi/full/10.1111/bjh.18083

Early-stage unfavourable criteria for cHL GHSG vs EORTC.

GHSG	EORTC
ESR ≥ 50 with no B-symptoms	ESR ≥ 50 with no B-symptoms
ESR ≥ 30 with B-symptoms	ESR ≥ 30 with B-symptoms
≥ 3 Lymph node sites	≥ 4 lymph node sites
Mediastinal: thoracic ratio of mass > 1/3 in diameter	Mediastinal: thoracic ratio of mass > 0.35 in diameter
Extranodal disease	Age ≥ 40

Hasenclever IPS score for assessing OS and PFS prediction.

Parameter	Score of 1
Age	≥ 45
Sex	Male
Albumin	< 40 g/L
Hb	< 105 g/L
WCC	$> 15 \times 10^9$/L
Lymphocyte count	$< 0.6 \times 10^9$/L

Total score	OS (%)
0–2	80–90%
2–4	60–80%
≥ 5	55%

Leukaemia

Acute Myeloid Leukaemia

Introduction: AML is an aggressive myeloid malignancy which can be novo or progress from other myeloproliferative/myelodysplastic conditions such as PRV, CML or CMML. The life-threatening subtype APML should always be screened for in AML diagnostics.

Epidemiology: 30–40% of all leukaemias with cure rate between 30–50% depending on risk stratification. Higher incidence in over 50's but can affect any age. Slight male predominance.

Signs/symptoms: Symptomatology often over weeks or a month or so. Lethargy, SOB, B-symptoms, infections, bleeding, pancytopenia, raised neutrophil count causing symptoms of hyperviscosity, rarely chloromas of skin can be at presentation.

FBC: Pancytopenia. If disease has spilled out into PB from BM may have a high count or if transformed from MPN or CML.

Blood film: Anaemia, thrombocytopaenia and neutropaenia. Circulating myeloid blasts. Assess myeloid series for sign of transformation from MDS or MPN. Bilobed blasts stacked with Auer rods = Faggot cell, which is typical of APML and should prompt urgent cytogenetics and initiation of ATRA.

Diagnosis: > 20% myeloid blasts in the PB or BM. Myeloid blasts < 20% with a recognised chromosomal translocation irrespective of percentage i.e., t(8;21), t(15;17), t(16;6) or inversion 16.

Flow panel: Useful for MRD monitoring and subtyping AML. Variation between subtypes. Common markers below.

Pos: CD13, 33, 34, 117, MPO and HLA-DR in most cases.

Neg: CD2, 3,10, 16, 19, 20, 22, 41, 61, TDT.

APML: CD 13, 33, 34, 117, MPO +ve, CD15 and HLA-DR -ve.

Subtyping: ELN for cytogenetics and molecular prognostication, WHO now splits AML by differentiation or by defining genetic abnormalities. WHO criteria by differentiation can be seen overleaf.

New WHO AML distinct molecular mutational subtypes include:
AML with *CEPBA* mutation.
AML with *KMT2A* rearrangement.
AML with *MECOM* rearrangement.
AML with *NUP98* rearrangement.
AML with *NPM1* mutation.
AML with *BCR::ABL1* fusion.
AML with *RUNX1::RUNXT1* fusion.
AML with *CBFB-MYH11* fusion.
AML with *DEK-NUP214* fusion.
AML with *RBM15:MRTFA* fusion.

The other distinct molecular subtypes not mentioned can be found below. Other WHO subtypes include, treatment related, AML NOS, AML with myelodysplastic related changes, related to Down syndrome, myeloid sarcoma or BPDCN.

Bone marrow: Flow panel as above with maturation arrest and myeloid blasts > 20%.

Cytogenetics: Useful for risk stratification and deciding on the need for an allograft.

Common translocations: t(15;17) (*PML-RARA*), inv16(*CBFB-MYH11*), t(8;21) (*RUNX1-RUNX1T1*) t(9;11) (*MLLT3-KMT2A*) t(;9:22) (*BCR-ABL1*) t(6:9) (*DEK-NUP214*). Deletions or inversions of chromosomes 3, 5, 7, 17 associated with poor risk disease.

Molecular: *FLT3* mutated in 1/3 of AML patients. Either ITD or TKD. Poor prognostic sign. Can treat with FLT3 inhibitor i.e., Midostaurin or gilteritinib. Can use as MRD marker. *NPM1* mutated in 30%. Good prognostic sign. In combination with *FLT3+* intermediate. Can use as MRD marker. *CEBPA* mutated in 8%. Good prognostic sign in biallelic mutations. *FLT3+* intermediate. Can use as MRD marker.

Tx at diagnosis? Yes, unless too old or frail for treatment and then best supportive care.

Other important work up: ECHO, G6PD, virology, tissue typing, PICC line, fertility counselling, CMV status pre-allo.

First line tx options: Split into transplant eligible vs ineligible based on fitness and AML subtype.

DA: (3+10 then 3+8) +/- FLT3 inhibitor +/- gemtuzumab (if CD33+ and no high-risk features) 2 cycles. Consolidate with 2 HiDAC or 2 DA.

FLAG IDA: Considered up front in high-risk disease though usually reserved for second line.

Aza/Ven: Non-intense regime. Can give until disease progression or intolerable toxicity. If not in CR after 2 cycles to consider change of treatment. ORR 70%.

Vyxeos: Liposomal DA with better side effects in secondary AML or therapy related AML.

APML: ATRA and ATO if WCC < 10 ATRA and AIDA if WCC > 10.

Elderly or frail: Single agent Azacitidine, hydroxycarbamide or low dose Ara-C. Consider best supportive care.

Emergency scenarios: Coagulopathy in APML. Leukostasis if blast count > 50×10^9/L. Neutropaenic sepsis.

Second/third line: FLAG-IDA or Aza/Ven if not tried initially. Clinical trial. Best supportive or palliative care.

Assessment of response: CR: < 5% blast in BM with recovery. PR: 5–25% blasts and > 50% reduction. RD: > 25% blasts.

Transplant: Poor risk in CR1. NPM1 +ve by MRD after second DA. Any risk CR2. Intermediate risk then consider an allo in CR1 or any time once CR achieved. Favourable risk in CR1 then no indication for transplant and reserved for relapsed disease.

Important side effects of tx: Severe neutropenic sepsis. Mucositis. Cardiac complications. TLS. ATRA differentiation syndrome in APML.

Supportive care: PCP, antiviral, bacterial and fungal prophylaxis, TLS, conjunctivitis from cytarabine, mouthwashes. Consider leukapheresis in high count presentation.

Trials to quote: PETHEMA group: Use of ATRA and Idarubicin in APML. VIALE-A: Aza/Ven in AML.

Other considerations: APML monitoring with marrows every 3/12 for 3 years.

Guidelines:
https://rmpartners.nhs.uk/wp-content/uploads/2020/01/Pan-London-AML-Guidelines-Jan-2020.pdf

AML European leukaemic network (ELN) risk stratification.

Genetic risk subtype	Cytogenetic/molecular abnormality	1-year OS
Favourable	Inversion or t(16;16) *CBFB-MYH11* t(8;21) *RUNX1* mutations t(15;17) *PML-RARA* *NPM1* mutation without *FLT3* *NPM1* mutation with low allelic burden ITD *FLT3* mutation Biallelic mutation of *CEPBA*	50–70%
Intermediate	t(9;11) *MLLT3-KMT2A* Mutated *FLT3* and *NPM1* Unmutated *FLT3* and *NPM1* Unmutated *NPM1* with low allelic burden ITD *FLT3* mutation Cytogenetic abnormality not falling into favourable or poor risk	40–50%
Poor	Inversion 3 or abnormal 3q. *GATA2* or *MECOM* mutation Deletion or additional 5, 5q, 7 or 7q 17p deletion or mutation. *TP53* t(11q23) t(6;9) *DEK-NUP214* t(9;22) *BCR-ABL* *KMT2A* rearranged with chromosome 6 or 10 *FLT3* mutation and *NPM1* unmutated Monosomal or Complex karyotype with ≥ 4 abnormalities Mutations in *ASXL1, RUNX1, EZH2, BCOR, SF3B1, SRSF2, c-KIT, STAG2 U2AF1* and *ZRSR2*	15–20%

WHO subtype of AML by differentiation.

AML classification	Positive flow markers
AML with minimal differentiation	CD13, 33, 34, 38, 117 HLA-DR and TdT
AML without maturation	CD7, 11b, 13, 33, 34, 117, HLA-DR and MPO
AML with maturation	CD7, 11b, 13, 15, 33, 34, 65, 117 and HLA-DR
Acute myelomonocytic leukaemia	CD7, 34, 117, HLA-DR. CD13, 15, 33 all variable Monocytes express: CD4, 11b, 11c, 14, 36, 64, 68 and 163.
Acute monocytic leukaemia	CD4, 11b, 11c, 13, 14, 15, 33, 34, 64, 65, 68, 117, HLA-DR and MPO
Acute erythroid leukaemia	CD36, 71, 117 and e-cadherin. CD34 negative
Acute megakaryoblastic leukaemia	CD13, 33, 36, 41, 42b, 61. CD7 variable

Chronic Myeloid Leukaemia

Introduction: CML is an MPN characterised by t(8;21) forming the BCR-ABL1 fusion gene termed the Philadelphia chromosome.

Epidemiology: 15–20% of leukaemias. 1.5:100,000. Radiation exposure may increase risk. 50-years-old there is a higher incidence but can affect any age. Slight male predominance.

Signs/symptoms: Asymptomatic (30%), constitutional symptoms i.e. fatigue or weight loss, splenomegaly, anaemia, bleeding, infection.

FBC: Neutrophilia, thrombocytosis and occasionally basophilia. Thrombocytopaenia or anaemia may suggest AP or BP.

Blood film: Left shift in myeloid series with all stages of maturation. Peak of neutrophils and myelocytes. Basophilia and blasts.

Diagnosis: PB and BM findings with BCR-ABL detected via PCR. Cytogenetic abnormalities, FBC indices, symptoms and blast % aid in diagnosis of AP or BP. ELN[1] vs WHO[2] criteria vary in AP and BP.

CP: < 10% blasts in PB or BM.

AP: 1 of: Basophils > 19% in PB, additional Ph+, clonal chromosome abnormalities or MRA, thrombocytopaenia < 100 × 10^9/L[1] or thrombocytosis > 1000 × 10^9/L[2], blasts > 15–29%[1] or 10–19% in PB/BM, increasing spleen or WCC on treatment[2].

BP: 1 of: PB/BM blasts > 29%[1] or >19%[2], Extramedullary blast infiltration, large cluster of blasts in BM[2].

Flow panel: Not useful in establishing diagnosis of CML. Can help quantify the number of myeloid blasts.

Stratification: 4 scores. Sokal, ELTS (Age, spleen, platelets, Pb blasts), Hasford (ELTS+ PB basophils and eosinophils), EUTOS.

Bone marrow: Hypercellular with myeloid hyperplasia. Raised M:E ratio. Packed marrow.

Cytogenetics/molecular: Major route abnormalities: trisomy 8 or 19, additional Ph+, isochrome 17q- all equate to poor OS.

Minor route abnormalities: del 7, 17, Y. gain of 17 or 21 and t(3;21).

Tx at diagnosis? Yes.

Other important work up: ECHO, G6PD, virology, tissue typing, PICC line, fertility preservation.

First line tx options: TKI but which one? TKI's like Nilotinib may improve time to MMR but not the rate of MMR achieved compared to traditional TKI imatinib. Use beneficial in those you want to get in MMR quickly. Imatinib, dasatinib and nilotinib approved for first line use. Consider 2G TKI if higher risk features or AP. Consider swapping to 3G TKI if BCR-ABL not < 10% by 3 months or if resistance mutation development. Treat BP as AML with second generation TKI alongside DA chemotherapy. *T315I* mutation then use Ponatinib or Asciminib (highly selective allosteric inhibitor).

Emergency scenarios: Leukostasis: WCC > 100 × 10⁹/L. HU 2–4 g/day and if needed leukapheresis. Beware TLS.

Second/third line: Those who fail imatinib should have tissue typing for allo and switch to 2G (dasatinib, nilotinib, bosutinib) or 3G based on side effect profile. Asciminib highly selective TKI used in *T315I* mutation. Consider clinical trial.

Assessment of response: BCR-ABL transcript monitored every 3 months. Goal is MMR or better at 1 year. Increase monitoring if warning signs from BCR-ABL transcript. Send mutation analysis in rising BCR-ABL transcript or treatment change.

Transplant: BP in CR as response to TKI alone transient. Secondary AP. AP treated with 2G not achieving MMR.

Important side effects of tx:

Imatinib: Muscle cramps, oedema, abnormal LFTs, CCF exacerbation.

Bosutinib: GI Bleeding, Abnormal LFTs, nausea and GI side effects.

Dasatinib: CCF exacerbation, pleural effusions, pulmonary HTN, GI bleeding.

Nilotinib: Thrombosis, HTN, CCF exacerbation and prolonged QT, abnormal blood sugars.

Ponatinib: Rash, thrombosis, HTN, raised lipids.

Asciminib: HTN, thrombosis, pancreatitis, rash.

Supportive care: Antiviral prophylaxis and consider antibacterial. Analgesia for splenomegaly. Allopurinol in high count.

Follow up: 3 monthly BCR-ABL. Weekly FBC for first month of treatment. BMAT every 3 months in those who fail TKI. Cessation of TKI if: CP only, TKI for 3–5 years, typical transcript, MMR4 (< 0.01%) for 2 years and no TKI resistance mutation.

4 weekly monitoring for 6 months, 6 weekly for 6 months, 2 monthly for 1 year, 3 monthly thereafter. If loss of MMR to resume TKI.

Trials to quote: German CML IV: Worse outcome of MRA. SPIRIT: TKI discontinuation. ASCEMBL: Use of Asciminib in CML.

Other considerations: TKI withdrawal syndrome: MSK pain following cessation. Basic analgesia, rheum review and trial of steroid.

Guidelines:

https://rmpartners.nhs.uk/wp-content/uploads/2020/01/Pan-London-CML-Guidelines-Jan-2020.pdf

https://onlinelibrary.wiley.com/doi/10.1111/bjh.16971

WHO vs ELN for staging.

Stage	Criteria	WHO	ELN
Chronic phase		Not fulfilling AP or BP	Not fulfilling AP or BP
Accelerated phase	Blast percentage	Blasts in PB or BM 10–19%	Blasts in PB or BM 15–29% OR Blasts < 30% but combined with promyelocytes > 30%
	Basophil percentage	$\geq$ 20% in PB	$\geq$ 20% in PB
	Platelets	Thrombocytopaenia < 100 × 10^9/ or Thrombocytosis > 1000 × 10^9/L unresponsive to treatment	Thrombocytopaenia < 100 × 10^9/L not treatment related
	Clinical	Increasing WCC or spleen size resistant to treatment	
	Chromosomal	New chromosomal abnormalities on treatment	New chromosomal or major route abnormalities on treatment
Blast phase	Blast percentage	Blasts in PB or BM $\geq$ 30%	Blasts in PB or BM $\geq$ 20%
	Clinical	Extramedullary blast proliferation in an organ other than the spleen	Extramedullary blast proliferation in an organ other than the spleen
	Bone marrow biopsy	Clusters of blasts in the bone marrow	

Targets for MRD monitoring of transcript and indications for switching TKI.

MRD interval	Target response	Warning signs	Treatment failure
Baseline	BCR-ABL ≤ 10%	No signs of haematological response or high-risk features of disease	
3 months	BCR-ABL ≤ 10%	BCR-ABL > 10%	No complete haematological response or new chromosomal abnormalities or mutations. Ph+ cells > 95%
6 months	BCR-ABL ≤ 10%	BCR-ABL ≤ 10% Ph+ cells 35–65%	BCR-ABL > 10% Ph+ cells > 65% New chromosomal abnormalities or mutations
12 months	BCR-ABL ≤ 1%	BCR-ABL 1–10% Ph+ cells 1–35%	BCR-ABL > 10% Ph+ cells > 35% New chromosomal abnormalities or mutations
Any time after 12 months	BCR-ABL ≤ 0.1%	BCR-ABL > 0.1% 2 consecutive chromosomal abnormalities showing chromosome 7 or 7q deletion	Loss of CHR or MMR New chromosomal abnormalities or mutations

Acute Lymphoblastic Leukaemia

Introduction: ALL is an aggressive but curable leukaemia of T and B-cells predominantly affecting children or adolescents.

Epidemiology: 15% of leukaemias, better outcomes in children than adults.

Signs/symptoms: Symptomatology often over weeks or short months. Lethargy, SOB, infections, bleeding, pancytopenia, raised lymphocyte count in high count disease, lymphadenopathy, splenomegaly, neurological manifestations, pleural effusions.

FBC: Lymphocytosis. Unlike AML not always maturation arrest though pancytopaenia commonly seen.

Blood film: Lymphocytosis +/- cytopaenias. Lymphoblasts seen. Agranular. May have cytoplasmic projections.

Diagnosis: 20% blasts or more in PB or BM.

Flow panel: Variation based on cell of origin precursor state.

B-ALL: **Pos:** CD10, 19, 22, 34, 79a, TdT. **Neg:** CD45, CD117.

T-ALL: **Pos:** TDT, cytoplasmic or surface CD3, CD7. **Neg:** CD8, 11c, 19, 20, 22. CD1a.

Subtyping:

B-ALL: Early Pre-B: CD10-. Pre-B: HLA-DR and cyIgM+. Mature B: sIgM+.

T-ALL: *Cortical T-ALL*: CD1a+. *Early T-ALL*: CD2 or 5+. *ETP-ALL*: 1 or more +ve myeloid/ stem cell markers.

Bone marrow: 20% blasts or more with or without maturation arrest.

Cytogenetics/molecular: *IgH* and *TCR* rearrangements used in MRD monitoring. Other rearrangements include t(12;21) (*TEL-AML1*), t(5;14) (*IL3-IGH*), t(1;19) (*E2A-PBX1*). See table below for WHO updates on classifying all B-ALL subtypes based on molecular mutations.

High risk abnormalities: Ph+, *IAMP21*, t(17;19), *MLL* rearranged and low hypodiploidy/ near triploidy.

Other important work up: ECHO, G6PD, virology, tissue typing, PICC line, fertility preservation. CMV status pre-allo. LP. CTNCAP in T-ALL and B-ALL if symptoms of concern such as LN or pain.

Tx at diagnosis? Yes.

First line tx options: Focusing on UKALL14 below. 2× induction, intensification, 4× consolidation, maintenance.

UKALL19: For 18–25-year-olds and Ph-.

UKALL60: > 60-years-old or not fit for SACT. Ph+ get imatinib throughout treatment phases.

UKALL14 (B-ALL): Induction 1 = Daunorubicin, vincristine, dexamethasone, asparaginase. IT-MTX(×2) +/- Rituximab.

UKALL14 (B-ALL): Induction 2 = Cyclophosphamide, cytarabine, mercaptopurine and IT-MTX(×4).

UKALL14 (T-ALL): Induction 2 = As above plus nelarabine.

UKALL14 (B-ALL): Intensification = IV MTX and asparaginase.

UKALL14 (B-ALL): C1 = Cytarabine, etoposide, asparaginase, IT MTX. C2 = Cytarabine, etoposide, IT MTX. C3 = Induction 1 + cyclophosphamide, cytarabine and 6MP. C4 = Cytarabine, etoposide, IT-MTX.

UKALL14 (B-ALL): Maintenance for 2 years = 3 monthly IT MTX, vincristine and prednisolone, 6MP daily, oral MTX weekly.

Emergency scenarios: CNS disease: IT MTX until CSF MRD -ve, generally on 2 consecutive samples.

Second/third line:

B-ALL: Blinatumomab (CD19+ bispecific antibody) or inotuzumab (CD22+ drug-antibody conjugate) in Ph-. Increased rates of VOD in latter post HSCT.

CAR-T: Considered at this point but eligible after 2nd line failure. Kymriah for < 25-years old, Yescarta for > 25 years-old.

T-ALL: Nelarabine or if Ph+ use a 2G TKI. Ponatinib licenced. Dasatinib crosses BBB.

CNS disease: HD MTX regime like MATRIX.

Clinical trials or palliative care should always be considered at relapse or if refractory.

Assessment of response: Nothing specific but usually marrow or CT after each cycle. Use of MRD monitoring if MRD marker positive.

Transplant: Done after induction or intensification. If ineligible proceed to consolidation. 25–65-year-olds consider at diagnosis. Other indications include Ph+, > 40-years-old, WCC > 30 (B-ALL) > 100 (T-ALL), MLL rearranged, Ho-Tr, complex karyotype, persistent MRD after induction 1, high risk cytogenetics in CR1, any relapse.

Important side effects of tx: Asparaginase: Risk of thrombosis. MTX: Renal dysfunction and mucositis. Nelarabine: Neurotoxicity.

Other consideration: PCP prophylaxis (not septrin due to MTX interaction). TLS in bulky nodal disease or high count.

Supportive care: PCP, antiviral, bacterial and fungal prophylaxis, TLS, conjunctivitis from cytarabine, mouthwashes for MTX.

Trials to quote: UKALL14: Nelarabine/rituximab randomisation. UKALL60: Safety and tolerability of protocols in > 60.

Guidelines:

https://rmpartners.nhs.uk/wp-content/uploads/2020/01/Pan-London-ALL-Guidelines-Jan-2020.pdf

http://www.ctc.ucl.ac.uk/TrialDocuments/Uploaded/UKALL14%20-%20Protocol%20-%20v5.0%202020.07.12%20plus%20errata%2004.02.14_12042017_0.pdf

New WHO B-ALL classification.

WHO new subtypes listed from updates in 2022	Old 2017 WHO terminology
B-ALL with *BCR::ABL1* fusion	B-ALL t(9;22), *BCR-ABL1*
B-ALL with *BCR::ABL1* like features	B-ALL, *BCR-ABL1* like
B-ALL high hyperdiploidy	B-ALL with hyperdiploidy
B-ALL with *KMT2A* rearrangement	B-ALL t(v11q23.3) *KMT2A* rearranged
B-ALL with *IGH::IL3* fusion	B-ALL with t(5;14) *IGH/IL3*
B-ALL with *TCF3::PBX1* fusion	B-ALL with t(1;19) *TCF3-PBX1*
B-ALL with *TCF3::HLF* fusion	Not included
B-ALL with *ETV6::RUNX1* fusion	B-ALL with t(12;21) *ETV6-RUNX1*
B-ALL with *ETV6::RUNX1* like features	Not included
B-ALL with other defined genetic abnormalities	Not included

In essence, the terminology has changed for most of them with a few new additions. Anything not falling into the new classification but with recognised B-ALL molecular mutation falls under B-ALL with other defined genetic abnormality.

Chronic Lymphocytic Leukaemia

Introduction: CLL is a clonal disorder of mature B-cells with differing prognostic groups based on cytogenic and molecular mutations.

Epidemiology: 25% of leukaemias and 3.5:100,000 new diagnosis each year. Median age 72. Male predominance.

Signs/symptoms: Often symptomless (50–70%), presenting following blood tests. B-symptoms, lymphadenopathy, splenomegaly, lethargy, autoimmune complications i.e., haemolysis or ITP.

FBC: Lymphocytosis +/- anaemia or thrombocytopenia depending on stage.

Blood film: Lymphocytosis of mature monomorphic lymphocytes with smear cells.

Diagnosis: > 5 × 10⁹/L Clonal B-lymphocytes. < 5 is MBL. < 5 with Lymph nodes is SLL.

Flow panel: CLL score > 3 suggestive of diagnosis. **Pos:** CD5, 19 and 23. Also now using CD200 bright. **Weak or neg:** CD22/79b, FMC7.

Bone marrow: Lymphocytosis often seen.

Lymph node Immunohistochemistry: Nil different from above.

Cytogenetics: 13q deletion, 17p deletion, 11q, trisomy 12, IgHV mutation.

Molecular: *TP53* and *IgHV* stratify risk. *SF3B1, CARD11, ATM* and *NOTCH* mutations among molecular panel which impact risk of RT.

Staging: Rai and Binet. Can also stage/risk stratify based on molecular mutations which also helps aid on treatment decisions. New staging strategies proposed based on molecular mutational burden recently published with 5 different subtypes and the risk they pose in progressive disease or Richter's transformation.

Tx at diagnosis? No.

Tx indications: <u>Based on International Working group CLL guidelines</u>: Symptomatic disease, Binet stage C disease, lymphocyte doubling time of < 3 months, intractable B symptoms, cytopaenias, painful splenomegaly or lymphadenopathy. If autoimmune complications — treat with steroids and consider CLL directed therapy if inadequate response.

Other important work up: ECHO, G6PD, virology, immunoglobulins, paraprotein, DAT, consider PET-CT if big bulky nodes to rule out RT.

First line tx options: Depending on *TP53* and appropriateness for chemotherapy. New NICE guidance that if FCR not suitable can use BTKi with ibrutinib and acalabrutinib licensed first line. Approach is BTKi vs O-Venetoclax or FCR though less commonly used. O-Venetoclax is a fixed duration therapy whereas BTKi is usually treat until progression. Patient choice and co-morbidities need to be considered. Fixed duration ibrutinib and Venetoclax also licensed.

Emergency scenarios: <u>Richter's transformation</u>: Progresses to high grade lymphoma protocol i.e., DLBCL.

Second/third line: Alternative BTKi vs chemoimmunotherapy vs R-Venetoclax if not used first line.

Third line or trial options: PI3K inhibitor vs consideration for allograft though there is a high TRM. Now the use of Ibrutinib-Venetoclax therapy NICE approved and superior outcome to O-Chlorambucil. Zanubrutinib still not NICE approved for CLL but FDA approved. Acalabrutinib is NICE approved.

Transplant: Not generally unless young and high risk/refractory disease. Consider after second/third tx failure.

Important side effects of tx: Tumour lysis syndrome in certain regimes, autoimmune complications of BTKi and cardiac arrythmias, risk of atypical severe infection with PI3K.

Supportive care: May need prophylactic antibiotics, monitor for TLS in high lymphocyte count with O-Venetoclax or with bulky nodal disease.

Trials to quote: Morono: O-Venetoclax use in CLL. CLL12: Ibrutinib vs placebo. CAPTIVATE: Fixed duration ibrutinib + venetoclax.

Other considerations: Irradiated blood products if previous FCR, vaccines, IV immuno-globulins if hypogammaglobulinemia and recurrent infections, empower patient to know baseline lymphocyte count.

Guidelines:

https://b-s-h.org.uk/guidelines/guidelines/guideline-for-the-treatment-of-chronic-lymphocytic-leukaemia/

https://rmpartners.nhs.uk/wp-content/uploads/2020/01/Pan-London-CLL-Guidelines-Jan-2020.pdf

Binet staging.

Stage	Disease characteristics
A	< 3 Lymph node groups affected
B	≥ 3 Lymph node group affected
C	Hb < 100g/L or platelets < 100 × 10^9/L

Rai staging.

Stage	Disease characteristics
0	Lymphocytosis
1	Lymphocytosis and lymphadenopathy
2	Lymphocytosis and splenomegaly
3/4	Lymphocytosis or lymphadenopathy and Hb < 110g/L or platelets < 100 × 10^9/L

Risk stratification based on molecular mutations.

Risk group	Molecular or cytogenetic mutation
Favourable	Mutated *IgHV* 13q deletion only No molecular mutations mentioned below
Unfavourable	17p deletion or mutations in *TP53* 11q or *ATM* mutations Trisomy 12 Unmutated *IgHV* Complex karyotype or high molecular mutational burden to genes such as *SF3B1, NOTCH1, BIRC3* CD38+ Treatment related mutations in genes such as *BTK* High ZAP70 expression

B-Prolymphocytic Leukaemia

B-PLL has now been removed from the WHO 2022 updates but at the time of writing was still included. For that reason, I have left it in for reference, but the entity no longer exists as per WHO classification.

Introduction: B-PLL is a rare aggressive leukaemia distinct from CLL.

Epidemiology: 1% of lymphoid leukaemias. Age of onset > 65. Slight male predominance. Extremely rare.

Signs/symptoms: Massive splenomegaly, high white cell count > 100×10^9/L, B-symptoms, anaemia and thrombocytopaenia.

FBC/Blood film: Smear cells, prolymphocytes and lymphocytes, anaemia and thrombocytopaenia.

Diagnosis: > 55% prolymphocytes in PB or on LN biopsy/BMAT.

Flow panel: Pos: CD19, 20, 22, FMC7, SmIg. **Weak:** Cd5, 79b +/-. **Neg:** CD23.

Bone marrow: Infiltration of prolymphocytes, often twice the size of lymphocytes with occasional nucleolus.

Cytogenetics: Common abnormalities include deletion 6q, 11q, 13q, 17p.

Molecular: *TP53* in 50% *c-MYC* in others.

Staging: As for CLL.

Tx at diagnosis? Nearly always yes. If no symptoms can watch and wait but regular close monitoring.

Other important work up: ECHO, G6PD, virology, immunoglobulins, HLA typing, PICC, fertility counselling based on treatment.

First line tx options: FCR or BR if not *TP53* mutated. BTKi if *TP53* mutation or alemtuzumab.

Second/third line: More intense regimes such as R-CHOP though CR not likely. Different BTKi if able to get funding. Splenectomy or splenic irradiation. Clinical trials.

Prognosis: Median OS 3 years.

Transplant: Allo in CR1 if suitable donor due to aggressive nature. Consider allo work up at diagnosis.

Important side effects of tx: As per CLL.

Supportive care: As per CLL.

Guidelines:
https://ashpublications.org/blood/article/120/3/538/30480/How-I-treat-prolymphocytic-leukemia

T-Prolymphocytic Leukaemia

Introduction: T-PLL is a very rare aggressive leukaemia distinct form CLL of mature T-cells.

Epidemiology: < 1% of lymphoid leukaemias but 33% of all T-cell malignancies. Age of onset > 60. Male predominance.

Signs/symptoms: Splenomegaly, lymphadenopathy, maculopapular rash, high white cell count often > 100, pleural effusions, anaemia or thrombocytopaenia.

FBC/Blood film: Prolymphocytes with cytoplasmic blebs.

Diagnosis: > 5 × 10⁹/L cells by flow or T-cell clonality and certain cytogenetic/molecular abnormalities as below.

Flow panel: Pos: CD2, 3, 5, 7. **Weak:** CD4, 8, 25, 52 +/-. **Neg:** Cd1a, TDT and B-cell markers.

Bone marrow: Infiltration of prolymphocytes as described above on film.

Cytogenetics: Common abnormalities include translocation or inversion 14. Isochrome 8q and complex karyotype.

Molecular: TCR rearrangements, mutations in *TCL-1*, *MTCP1*, *ATM* genes commonly, altered telomer lengths reported.

Staging: <u>Active disease</u>: B-symptoms, BM failure, LN or splenic disease, doubling time, extranodal disease.

Tx at diagnosis? Nearly always yes. If no symptoms can watch and wait but regular close monitoring required. Most would treat at diagnosis.

Other important work up: ECHO, G6PD, virology, immunoglobulins, HLA typing, PICC, fertility based on treatment. HTLV1 as part of differential work up for AITL.

First line tx options: Alemtuzumab, achieve CR1 then allograft if donor or autograft if not. Campath (anti-CD52 monoclonal antibody).

Second/third line: Pentostatin if not in CR. Nelarabine or clinical trial if failure on second line.

Prognosis: Median OS 2–3 years.

Important side effects of tx: Alemtuzumab reactions and fever.

Supportive care: As per CLL.

Guidelines:
https://ashpublications.org/blood/article/120/3/538/30480/How-I-treat-prolymphocytic-leukemia

Hairy Cell Leukaemia

Introduction: HCL is a rare B-cell leukaemia characterised by lymphocytes with long thin villous projection, characteristic flow panel and monocyotpaenia.

Epidemiology: < 1% of all leukaemias. 2% of lymphoid leukaemias. Good 5-year OS of 90–95%. Peak age of onset is 55–60. Male predominance.

Signs/symptoms: Asymptomatic in some. Hepatosplenomegaly, lethargy, bleeding, infection, pancytopenia and monocyotpaenia. Leucocytosis in HCL-V and no mono-cyotpaenia. Lymphadenopathy in around 10%.

FBC/film: Lymphocytes with finger-like "hairy" cytoplasmic projections and oval nucleus without nucleolus.

Diagnosis: HCL score from flow cytometry of ≥ 3 and presence of cells morphologically. IHC positive from BM for CD20 and Cyclin D1+. *BRAF V600E* mutated as is *SOX11*.

Flow panel: Score of 3 or more suggestive of diagnosis. **Pos:** Cd11c, 25, 103, 123. **Other pos:** CD20. **Variable expression:** CD27, 43, 81, 200. **Neg:** CD27 and 38 in HCL compared to HCL-V.

Subtyping: HCL-V shows prominent nucleoli, CD25 and 123 -ve, CD27+.

Bone marrow: Often a dry tap due to fibrosis from HCL infiltrate. Hypocellular and "fried egg" morphology on H and E stain.

Molecular: HCL: Mutated *BRAF* in almost 100%. HCL-V: *MAP2K1* gene mutations.

Tx at diagnosis? Yes.

Other important work up: ECHO, G6PD, virology, PICC line, fertility preservation, CT staging if lymphadenopathy.

First line tx options: Cladribine or pentostatin with an ORR of 90–100%. Long remissions expected.

Pentostatin: Injection every 3 weeks until in remission.

Cladribine: IV or SC infusion.

HCL-V treatment: Pentostatin is inferior in HCL-V. Cladribine-Rituximab instead. MAP2K inhibitors also used if mutated.

Emergency scenarios: Severe infection due to pancytopaenia. Nil else disease related. No TLS unless bulky LN.

Second/third line: 50% will relapse despite good ORR.

Options: Consider repeat R-cladribine if good PFS from 1st line. R-benda, moxetumomab (CD22 antibody-conjugate), BRAF inhibitors (vemurafenib), BTKi and clinical trials.

Assessment of response: BMAT after 4–6 months of treatment.

CR: No hairy cells in PB/BM and resolution of organomegaly/lymphadenopathy.

PR: 50% resolution of above and no cytopaenias.

Transplant: No role unless multiple relapsed resistant disease and donor or HCL-V without response to treatment.

Important side effects of tx: <u>Pentostatin</u>: Long term nausea post injection. <u>Cladribine</u>: Widespread erythrodermic rash.

Other consideration: Irradiated products following cladribine.

Supportive care: GCSF for pancytopaenia if prolonged. PCP, antiviral and antibacterial prophylaxis.

Guidelines:

https://onlinelibrary.wiley.com/doi/10.1111/bjh.17055

Large Granular Lymphocytic Leukaemia

Introduction: Rare lymphoid leukaemia which is T or NK-cell subtype with increase in LGL cells in PB.

Epidemiology: < 1:1,000,000 people. Extremely rare.

T-LGL: Median age of onset 60 or younger in aggressive disease.

NK-Cell: Aggressive and mild forms exist. Aggressive form has a very poor prognosis. EBV associated.

Signs/symptoms:

T-LGL: Asymptomatic, lymphocytosis, neutropaenia, fatigue or immune symptoms, splenomegaly, cytopaenias, LN, B-symptoms.

NK-LGL: Largely asymptomatic with mild neutropaenia.

FBC/Blood film: Lymphocytes with azurophilic granules in abundant blue cytoplasm and eccentric nucleus.

Diagnosis: Clonal LGL population with mature T or NK-cell flow phenotype. No specific threshold.

Flow panel:

T-LGL: **Pos:** CD3, 8, 16, 57. **Weak or variants:** CD4, 5, 7, 8. **Neg:** CD56, TdT.

T-LGL aggressive form: **Pos:** CD3, 8, 56. **Neg:** CD57, TdT.

NK-LGL: **Pos:** CD2, 11b, 16, 56. **Weak or variants:** CD57. **Neg:** CD3, 4, 7 ,8, TDT.

Bone marrow: As for blood film with nodular or diffuse infiltrate.

Cytogenetics: Rearrangement of TCR genes. Marker of clonality and can be used for assessing MRD.

Molecular: *STAT3* mutations common.

Staging: Chronic NK: Asymptomatic with flow pattern.

Aggressive: Symptoms with flow pattern.

Tx at diagnosis? Yes, in aggressive disease. Indications for treatment include infection, symptoms or bone marrow infiltration i.e., anaemia or thrombocytopaenia.

Other important work up: ECHO, G6PD, virology, immunoglobulins, HLA typing in NK aggressive form.

First line tx options:

NK and indolent T-LGL: Low dose MTX, ciclosporin or cyclophosphamide. Steroids for neutropaenia.

Aggressive T-LGL: ALL regime such as UKALL14 with CNS prophylaxis.

Second/third line:

NK and indolent T-LGL: Alemtuzumab or purine analogues, STAT3 inhibitors, CHOP regimes, trials.

Aggressive T-LGL: Clinical trial.

Prognosis:
NK and indolent T-LGL: Not curable but good median OS of 9–10 years.
Aggressive T-LGL: As little as 2–3 months if no transplant. Even with allograft median OS 2 years.
Transplant: In aggressive T and NK forms allograft in CR1.
Important side effects of Tx: Irradiated products after purine analogues. MTX side effects i.e., mucositis. UKALL14 side effect profile. Haemorrhagic cystitis with cyclophosphamide. Ciclosporin toxicity.
Supportive care: Antibiotics for infection, GCSF for neutropaenia and infection prevention.
Guidelines:
https://www.lls.org/leukemia/large-granular-lymphocytic-leukemia
https://rmpartners.nhs.uk/wp-content/uploads/2020/01/Pan-London-Less-Common-Guidelines-Jan-2020.pdf

Adult T-Cell Leukaemia/Lymphoma

Introduction: Rare aggressive mature T-cell leukaemia associated with HTLV-1 infection of CD4+ cells.

Epidemiology: Rare. Of the 20 million infected with HTLV-1 worldwide only 1–5% develop ATLL. Higher in Afro-Caribbean and Southeast Asian populations. Any age based on length of time of infection. Median age 58. Slight male predominance.

Signs/symptoms: Hypercalcaemia, elevated WCC, rashes, hepatosplenomegaly, lymphadenopathy, fevers, atypical infections.

FBC/Blood film: WCC > 500 $\times$ 10⁹/L in acute form, anaemia and thrombocytopaenia. Lobulated clover leaf nucleus lymphocyte.

Diagnosis: HTLV1+ with clonal T lymphocytes in PB/LN/BM with characteristic flow pattern.

<u>Smouldering</u>: Normal lymphocyte count but ATL cells seen on PB between 1–5%, no organomegaly or LN, normal calcium, occasional skin/lung lesions.

<u>Chronic</u>: Lymphocyte count > 4 $\times$ 10⁹ $\times$ 10⁹/L, enlarged LN, organomegaly, mild skin involvement, normal calcium.

<u>Acute</u>: Lymphocyte count > 4 $\times$ 10 $\times$ 10⁹/L⁹ with high percentage of ATLL cells, maturation arrest, pleural effusions, abdominal pain, LN, organomegaly, large skin lesion, hypercalcaemia, raised LDH.

<u>Lymphomatous</u>: < 1% circulating ATL cells large bulky LN, few circulating ATL cells, Raised LDH, probable hypercalcaemia.

Flow panel: Pos: CD2, 3, 4, 5, 25, HTLV1+, HLADR+. **Neg:** TdT, CD 7, 8, 16, 56.

Bone marrow: Diffuse infiltration with ATL cells with characteristic flow pattern.

Cytogenetics: TCR clonality and gene rearrangement, gain of chromosome 3 and 7, deletion 13. Vary depending on subtype generally.

Molecular: *TLSC1* expression, *TP53* mutation in a third.

Staging: <u>Order of prevalence</u>: Acute/leukaemic, chronic, lymphomatous and smouldering.

Tx at diagnosis? Yes, in acute or lymphomatous disease. Close observation in chronic or smouldering can be done.

Other important work up: ECHO, G6PD, virology, immunoglobulins, HLA typing, PICC, fertility counselling based on treatment, strongyloides serology as risk of co-infection with HTLV-1. Provide eradication therapy if +ve prior or during treatment.

First line tx options: AZT and IFN in all subtypes except lymphomatous. Add CHOP/CHOEP for lymphomatous +/- monoclonal antibody treatment with the CCR4 inhibitor mogamulizumab. Consider AZT and IFN maintenance while waiting for donor for allograft.

Second/third line: Trials, monoclonal antibodies.

Prognosis: Aggressive forms median OS < 1 year. Indolent or smouldering 2–4-year OS.

Transplant: Yes, in eligible patients in CR1.

Important side effects of tx: Osteonecrosis with AZT in prolonged exposure. Reactions with mogamulizumab.

Other consideration: CNS prophylaxis to consider.

Supportive care: Antiviral, antifungal and antibacterial prophylaxis, check immuno-globulins, PCP prophylaxis, Strongyloides eradication and GCSF for severe neutropaenia.

Guidelines:

https://b-s-h.org.uk/media/2895/t-nhl-guideline-3-8-13-updated-with-changes-accepted-v1-rg.pdf/

https://acsjournals.onlinelibrary.wiley.com/doi/full/10.1002/cncr.32556#:~:text=Globally%2C%205%20million%20to%2010,can%20be%20challenging%20to%20diagnose

https://rmpartners.nhs.uk/wp-content/uploads/2020/01/Pan-London-Less-Common-Guidelines-Jan-2020.pdf

Myeloproliferative Disorders

Essential Thrombocytosis

Introduction: ET is a chronic clonal myeloproliferative disorder associated with specific molecular mutations and thrombocytosis.

Epidemiology: Affects 1:35,000. Affects elderly more commonly. Median age 60. No sex predominance.

Signs/symptoms: Often asymptomatic. Those with symptoms are often thrombo-haemorrhagic. Pruritis also.

FBC/Blood film: Thrombocytosis, if progressing to MF or AML then may see associated changes on film. No blasts in ET.

Diagnosis:

- Platelet count > 450 × 10⁹/L with no reactive cause.
- Associated molecular mutation of *JAK2*, *CALR* or *MPL* without other underlying haematological malignancy.
  Or if no disease defining molecular mutation
- BMAT with increased megakaryopoesis and characteristic of ET.

Bone marrow: Performed to rule out pre-existing conditions, such as pre-fibrotic MF. Shows increase in hyperlobulated megakaryocytes.

Cytogenetics/Molecular: *JAK2* most common, *CALR* next then *MPL*. 15% may have other molecular mutation in myeloid gene panel.

Staging: BSH or IPSET staging for risk groups.

BSH: *Low*: < 40-years-old and no high-risk features. *Intermediate*: 40–60 and no high-risk features. *High*: > 60 or thrombosis.

IPSET score: *Low*: 0. *Intermediate*: 1–2. *High*: > 2. Factors: Age > 60, thrombosis, *JAK2 V617F* or vascular risk factors.

Tx at diagnosis? Depends on risk group. Generally low dose aspirin in all. Cytoreductive therapy in most. Target platelet count < 400 × 10⁹/L to reduce thrombo-haemorrhagic complications.

Other important work up: *JAK2 Exon 12* if the initial molecular is -ve though often done regardless now. Rule out other differentials: Iron panel, haematinics, autoimmune screen, infection screen, abdominal USS for splenomegaly, CXR, smoking history, *BCR-ABL* for CML. Consider VWF screen if bleeding + high count for acquired VWD.

First line tx options: Aspirin unless high platelet count or bleeding history. If age > 60 generally treat with cytoreductive therapy.

Intermediate/High risk: Cytoreductive therapy with hydroxycarbamide (HU) or pegylated interferon.

Second/third line: <u>High risk</u>: Hydroxycarbamide or pegylated interferon. Anagrelide. Busulphan. Clinical trial.

Prognosis: Very good. Most have OS of > 15 years.

Transplant: Consider allograft if transformation to MF or AML. Often have complex karyotype.

Important side effects: <u>HU</u>: Myelosuppression, sepsis, skin breaks or ulceration, hepatotoxicity, depression, secondary cancers.

Trials to quote: <u>MRC-PT1</u>: Addition of aspirin to HU in intermediate patients no benefit. <u>ANAHDRET</u>: Use of anagrelide.

Supportive care: Regular FBC for monitoring. Anticoagulation if thrombosis. Teratogenicity on HU. Monitor TFTs + LFTs on Interferon.

Other considerations: Rule out reactive cause. Transformation to Myelofibrosis or AML. Acquired VWD.

Guidelines:

https://onlinelibrary.wiley.com/doi/10.1111/bjh.17766

https://onlinelibrary.wiley.com/doi/full/10.1111/bjh.12986

https://rmpartners.nhs.uk/wp-content/uploads/2020/01/Pan-London-MPN-Guidelines-Jan-2020.pdf

Polycythaemia Rubra Vera

Introduction: Chronic clonal erythrocytosis with myeloid molecular mutations and associated erythema, pruritis and thrombosis.

Epidemiology: Incidence of 1:45,000. Slight male predominance. More common in middle age/elderly. Median age 55–60.

Signs/symptoms: Many asymptomatic. Those with symptoms include pruritis, splenomegaly, thrombosis, hyperviscosity, gout.

FBC/Blood film: Erythrocytosis, packed red cells, occasionally thrombocytosis or neutrophilia.

Diagnosis: Can be *JAK2* +ve or *JAK2* -ve PRV. Can also perform red cell mass studies and *JAK2* exon 12 molecular if *JAK2 V617F* is -ve.

JAK2 +ve:

- Haematocrit > 0.52 in men or > 0.48 in women.
- JAK2 mutation.

JAK2 -ve: See table below.

Bone marrow: Useful if concerns for transformation to AML or *JAK2* -ve on molecular testing to reach a diagnosis. Shows increased erythropoiesis, granulopoiesis and megakaryopoesis with hyperlobulated forms. Helps rule our pre-fibrotic MF.

Cytogenetics/Molecular: *JAK2V617F* +ve in large majority of patients. *TET2* and *DNMT3A* reported in *JAK2* -ve cases. Transformation to MDS, MF or AML can occur and more likely in those with complex karyotype.

Staging:

Low: < 65-years-old + no thrombosis. High WCC or cardiovascular risk factors would make an individual in this group higher risk.

High: > 65-years-old or previous thrombosis.

Intermediate: Not fulfilling high or low risk criteria.

Tx at diagnosis? Depends on risk stratification but generally yes.

Other important work up: Rule out reactive causes: Smoking status, B12 and folate, alcohol history, serum erythropoietin level, USS for splenomegaly, sleep studies, lung function, consider further molecular testing for rare causes such as erythropoietin receptor mutations.

First line tx options: Goals of treatment are to reduce risk of splenomegaly, transformation to AML/MF/MDS or thrombosis. Aim for haematocrit < 0.45.

Low risk: Venesection to achieve target of < 0.45. Low dose aspirin.

High risk or symptomatic: Cytoreductive therapy with HU.

Second/third line: If intolerant or resistant to HU change to interferon-alpha, ruxolitonib, anagrelide, busulfan or clinical trial.

Prognosis: Often chronic and manageable in most. 5–10% risk of transformation to AML/MF/MDS.

Transplant: Allograft if transformation to AML, MF or MDS and fit enough.
Important side effects of tx: Myelosuppression, sepsis, skin breaks or ulceration, secondary cancers, anaemia.
Trials to quote: ECLAP study: Lead to risk stratification based on age. Higher chance of transformation if > 70-years-old.
Supportive care: Regular FBC for monitoring. Anticoagulation if thrombosis. Teratogenicity on HU. Monitor thyroid and liver function on Interferon.
Other considerations: Risk of stroke in high haematocrit.
Guidelines:
https://onlinelibrary.wiley.com/doi/10.1111/bjh.17766
https://onlinelibrary.wiley.com/doi/full/10.1111/bjh.12986
https://rmpartners.nhs.uk/wp-content/uploads/2020/01/Pan-London-MPN-Guidelines-Jan-2020.pdf

JAK2 -ve criteria for diagnosis of PRV requires all from absolute criteria and 1 from column B or 2 C.

Absolute criteria	Additional criteria column B	Additional criteria column C
Red cell mass > 25% or HCT > 0.6 in men and 0.56 in women	BM biopsy appearance of PRV	Platelet count > 450 × 10^9/L
JAK2 -ve	Splenomegaly on examination	Neutrophilia > 10 × 10^9/L (check smoking history as higher threshold of 12.5 × 10^9/L)
No obvious cause for reactive PRV identified	Absences of other myeloid associated molecular mutations such as CALR or BCR-ABL present	Splenomegaly on USS
		Low EPO level

Myelofibrosis

Introduction: BCR-ABL -ve MPN which exists as de novo, transformed from other MPN or pre-fibrotic subtypes.

Epidemiology: 1:100,000. Median age of onset 50–60. No sex predominance.

Signs/symptoms: B-symptoms, splenomegaly, cytopaenias, anaemia, thrombosis, lethargy, abdominal pain.

FBC/Blood film: Leukoerythroblastic blood film, tear drop red cells, blasts, nucleated red cells and left shifted.

Diagnosis:

- Bone marrow fibrosis.
- *BCR-ABL* -ve.
- Meeting WHO criteria below.

BSH criteria also exist which are largely similar though minor criteria include constitutional symptoms and extramedullary haematopoiesis and major criteria is bone marrow fibrosis ≥ grade 2.

Bone marrow: Hypercellular for age, staghorn megakaryocytes, reticulin deposition, erythroid hypoplasia.

Cytogenetics/Molecular: *ASXL1, EZH2, TET2, SF3B1* mutations common. Chromosome 3, 5, 7, 8 abnormalities indicate poor prognosis.

Grading: Based on severity of reticulin deposition in marrow and degree of osteosclerosis. Grade 0–3.

Staging: IPSS for diagnosis. DIPSS or DIPSS plus for follow up assessment. Based on age, Hb, blasts, WCC and B-symptoms.

Tx at diagnosis? Generally, yes unless low risk and poor performance status.

Other important work up: USS abdomen, *BCR-ABL*, LDH, myeloid gene panel, haematinics, exclude secondary causes.

First line tx options: Aims of treatment are to reduce symptoms of splenomegaly, prevent progression and prevent thrombosis. Aspirin in all patients. Ruxolitonib in symptomatic splenomegaly if risk is intermediate 2 or more. HU if not symptomatic/ low risk.

Second/third line: Ruxolitonib if not first line. Options include: Interferon, busulfan, azacitadine or LDAC in accelerated MF or worse. Trial.

Prognosis: Based on staging. Low risk median OS 10–12 years. High risk 2–3 years. Transformation to AML 25% chance in MF.

Transplant: Allograft if transformation or if high risk in CR1 using RIC. If refractory or progressive disease also consider allo.

Important side effects of tx: Ruxolitonib can cause myelosuppression. Needs close monitoring to assess response vs toxicity.

Trials to quote: <u>COMFORT-II trial</u>: JAK inhibitors improved OS.

Supportive care: Transfusion support. EPO to be considered. Anticoagulation for thrombotic complications.

Guidelines:
https://onlinelibrary.wiley.com/doi/full/10.1111/bjh.12985
https://rmpartners.nhs.uk/wp-content/uploads/2020/01/Pan-London-MPN-Guidelines-Jan-2020.pdf

WHO Pre-fibrotic MF criteria. Require all 3 major and 1 minor.

Major criteria	Minor criteria
JAK2, *CALR* or *MPL* mutation or if -ve another clonal mutation in a relevant gene such as *ASXL1*	Anaemia
Not meeting criteria for other MPN, Ph- CML or MDS	Splenomegaly on examination
BM biopsy shows atypical megakaryocytes, hypergranular with granulocytic proliferation, reduced erythropoiesis, BM fibrosis which is not grade 1	WCC > 11 × 10⁹/L
	Raised LDH

WHO Overt MF criteria. Require all 3 major and 1 minor.

Major criteria	Minor criteria
JAK2, *CALR* or *MPL* mutation or if -ve another clonal mutation in a relevant gene such as *ASXL1*	Anaemia
Not meeting criteria for other MPN, Ph- CML or MDS	Splenomegaly on examination
Megakaryocyte proliferation or atypical forms with grade 2 or more reticulin or collagen bone marrow fibrosis on biopsy	WCC > 11 × 10⁹/L
	Raised LDH
	Leucoerythroblastic blood film

IPSS

Parameter	Score of 1
Age	> 65
WCC (× 10⁹/L)	> 25
Hb	< 100*
% Blasts in PB	≥ 1%
B-Symptoms	Yes

Total score	Risk	Median OS
0	Low	Not yet reached
1–4	Intermediate	4 years
≥ 5	High	1.5 years

*Score of 2

Primary Eosinophilic Syndromes

Introduction: Clonal disorders of eosinophils without reactive cause, and numerous recognised gene rearrangements. When persisting without symptoms for greater than 6 months it can be classified as chronic eosinophilic leukaemia.

Epidemiology: Very rare. Affects any age. No sex predominance.

Signs/symptoms: Rash, pruritis, thrombosis, fevers, cytokine release syndromes, wheeze and SOB, chest pain.

FBC/Blood film: Eosinophilia seen with total eosinophil count $> 0.5 \times 10^9$/L.

Diagnosis: Eosinophilia $> 1.5 \times 10^9$/L and Symptoms should prompt investigation. If persistent for 6 months classify as chronic eosinophilic leukaemia. FISH or Rt-PCR should be used with bone marrow examination for diagnosis of primary eosinophilic syndrome.

Flow panel: Not used. **Bone marrow:** Eosinophilia typically $> 6\%$ on differential. Look for blasts or signs of LPD.

Cytogenetics/Molecular: *JAK2*, *c-KIT(KITD816V* mutation), *PDGFRA*, *PDGFRB*, *FIP1L1* or *FGFR1* mutations. *ETV6* translocations with *ABL1* and *FLT3*.

Tx at diagnosis? Yes, unless chronic eosinophilic leukaemia without symptoms, end organ damage and no gene rearrangements.

Other important work up: Rule out reactive causes: Strongyloides and flatworm serology, drug history, travel history autoimmune screen, assessment for end organ damage i.e., troponin. Other solid organ cancers or vasculitis. Lymphoproliferative disorders or CML. Mast cell tryptase should also be done.

First line tx options:

Imatinib: In *PDGFRA*, *PDGFRB* or *FIPL1L* rearrangements/mutations. Low dose is effective and MRD analysis can guide if able to stop.

Ruxolitonib: In *JAK2* mutations.

Sorafenib or sunitinib/other FLT3 inhibitor: *ETV6-FLT3* translocation. Consider clinical trial in all. *FGFR1* mutations not TKI sensitive.

Emergency scenario: End organ damage: Treat with high dose corticosteroids 1 mg/kg of methylprednisolone. Ivermectin if risk of Strongyloides.

Second/third line: Clinical trial. Other TKI or molecular targeted therapy. Allograft following high dose systemic chemotherapy.

Prognosis: *FGFR1* poor prognosis compared to other molecular abnormalities. Consider AML like treatment for these.

Transplant: Allograft in those who transform to AML or in those with *FGFR1* in CR1 or in those intolerant of treatment or relapsed/refractory disease.

Important side effects of tx: TKI side effects as mentioned in CML section.

Guidelines:

https://onlinelibrary.wiley.com/doi/full/10.1111/bjh.14488

Mast Cell Disorders

Introduction: Clonal neoplastic proliferation of mast cells often with elevated tryptase manifesting as systemic, cutaneous or sarcoma variants.
Incidence: Very rare. Affects any age. No sex predominance.
Signs/symptoms: Highly variable. Cutaneous manifestations with rashes. Systemic manifestations with urticaria, abdominal pain, GI symptoms, inflammatory syndromes, raised tryptase.
FBC/Blood film: Cytopaenias in mast cell leukaemia, increased population of mast cells.
Diagnosis: If tryptase > 20 ng/ml with symptoms investigate patients for mast cell disorders. Diagnostic criteria below.
Cutaneous: Skin only manifestations on biopsy. Most common form.
Systemic: Skin and end organ disease such as bone marrow or spleen. Indolent and aggressive forms.
SM-AHN: In older population, aggressive disease.
Mast cell leukaemia: Worst outcome with > 20% clonal mast cells in BM or > 10% PB.
Flow panel: CD117+.
Cytogenetics/Molecular: *c-KIT(KITD816V)* mutations in 90%. Others include *ASXL1*, *TET2* and other myeloid mutations.
Tx at diagnosis? Yes. Poor prognosis and hard to treat. Diagnosis often made late.
Other important work up: Serum tryptase, drug and allergy history, infective screen, autoimmune screen.
First line tx options: Always consider clinical trial if available.
Localised cutaneous: Local steroids or PUVA if resistant.
Systemic: *c-KIT* +ve: Midostaurin. *c-KIT* -ve: Dasatinib or imatinib.
Mast cell leukaemia: Midostaurin and DA chemotherapy.
Second/third line: Trial or interferon. Consider brentuximab if CD30+.
Prognosis: Varies based on subtype. Mast cell leukaemia poor prognosis.
Transplant: Allograft in CR1 of aggressive disease or in any relapse or treatment resistance where appropriate.
Supportive care: Analgesia, GI symptom control, antihistamines, hypotension management.
Important side effects of tx: TKI side effects. Angioedema from Midostaurin.
Guidelines:
https://onlinelibrary.wiley.com/doi/full/10.1111/bj0.14967

SM diagnostic criteria. 1 major and 1 minor required or 3 minor.

Major	Minor
BM biopsy showing islands or aggregates of mast cells.	*KIT816V* mutation
	Mast cells expressing CD2 and/or CD25
	Serum tryptase > 20 ng/ml
	> 25% atypical or spindle shaped mast cells on BM biopsy

B and C findings in addition to above for further classification.

B findings	C findings
> 30% mast cell infiltrate of cellularity on BM biopsy + serum tryptase > 200 ng/ml	Mast cell infiltrate and 1 or more cytopaenias
Dysplasia or proliferation in non-mast cells not satisfying other criteria for associated neoplasm	Palpable hepatosplenomegaly with organ impairment
Hepatosplenomegaly without organ impairment or lymphadenopathy	Splenomegaly with hypersplenism
	GI mast cell infiltrate and associated symptoms
	Lytic lesions

Classification of SM

1. <u>Systemic mastocytosis</u>: Meets SM diagnostic criteria without associated neoplasm.
2. <u>Systemic mastocytosis with associated haematological neoplasm</u>: Meets SM diagnostic criteria and associated neoplasm.
3. <u>Indolent systemic mastocytosis</u>: Meets SM criteria and no C findings and not meeting criteria for mast cell leukaemia or associated neoplasm.
4. <u>Smouldering systemic mastocytosis</u>: Meets SM criteria and no C findings but 2 or more B findings and no associated haematological neoplasm.
5. <u>Aggressive systemic mastocytosis</u>: Meets SM criteria, no evidence of mast cell leukaemia and 1 or more C finding.
6. <u>Mast cell leukaemia</u>: Meets SM criteria but BM biopsy ≥ 20% atypical mast cells with mast cell aggregates, often with ≥ 10% in PB.
7. <u>Mast cell sarcoma</u>: No SM criteria and biopsy showing mast cell infiltrate which is destructive and high grade.
8. <u>Cutaneous mastocytosis</u>: Not meeting any other criteria with limited skin disease proven on biopsy in either diffuse or limited forms or solitary mastocytoma of skin which is often low grade and non-destructive.

NOTE: *Think of the classification of these disorders a bit like MGUS, smouldering myeloma, myeloma, plasmacytomas etc.*

Plasma Cell Dyscrasias

Monoclonal Gammopathy of Undetermined Significance

Introduction: Pre-malignant monoclonal paraproteinemia with heterogeneous course that can progress to multiple myeloma.

Incidence/age: Higher incidence with age. 3% over 50-years-old affected. Risk of progression to MM 1% per year. Varying risk categories.

Signs/symptoms: Often asymptomatic, rarely bleeding or neuropathy. Lethargy or thrombosis sometimes but again rare. Raised ESR.

FBC/Blood film: Often nothing, maybe rouleaux.

Diagnosis:

- PP < 30 g/L.
- BMAT < 10% plasma cells.
- No signs or symptoms of MM or related lymphoplasmacytoid malignancies and urinary paraprotein < 500 mg/day.

Bone marrow: < 10% plasma cells. If greater than that becomes either asymptomatic/smouldering MM or MM.

Cytogenetics/molecular: As per MM for risk stratifying disease.

Subtypes: IgA or IgG progress to MM or amyloidosis. IgM progresses to WM. Light chain MGUS progresses to light chain MM.

Staging: Mayo MGUS risk stratification model deems high risk if: Non-IgG subtype, rapidly rising PP, PP > 15 g/L SFLC > 500 mg/L. abnormal SFLC ratio (< 0.26 or > 1.65 mg/L). High risk chance of progression to MM at 20 years 60% compared to 5% in low risk and 20–35% in intermediate.

Tx at diagnosis? No, monitor regularly every 3 months and if PP rising or new symptoms MRI or BMAT. Increase monitoring if rising. Low or low-intermediate risk does not require BMAT or imaging. Any other risk should be investigated with imaging and BM. Low or low-intermediate risk can be seen in primary care 6 months after diagnosis and then yearly after. Any other risk should be seen by haematology.

Other important work up: Albumin, B2M, urine Bence Jones protein, SFLC, calcium, MRI or other imaging to consider, BMAT, renal panel, LDH, blood film.

Emergency scenarios: Transformation to MM, amyloidosis, lymphoplasmacytoid malignancies or plasma cell leukaemia.

First line tx options: Monitoring in primary care if well, IgG < 15 or other subtype < 10. Refer if 25% rise and minimum 5 g/L in 3 months, new symptoms or lab findings suggesting progression to myeloma.

Prognosis: Risk of progressing to MM and dying in 20 years is 25% in high risk and 2% in low risk.

Transplant: Not unless transformed to MM then consider auto in first PR or better in those eligible.

Supportive care: Neuropathy management and renal monitoring.

Other considerations: MGRS: MGUS causing renal disease without criteria to meet myeloma. i.e., plasma cell percentage or SFLC not significant. B-cell clone is small. Always consider AL amyloidosis in these patients. Consider steroids or velcade containing regimes.

Guidelines:

https://onlinelibrary.wiley.com/doi/full/10.1111/j.1365-2141.2009.07807.x

https://www.kingshealthpartners.org/assets/000/003/349/Pan_London_Plasma_Cell_Guidelines_Jan_2020_original.pdf

Smouldering/Asymptomatic Myeloma

Introduction: MM diagnostic criteria met in respect to PP or plasma cell % without presence of end organ damage CRAB criteria.

Incidence/age: As above for MGUS. Higher rate of transformation to MM or other plasma cell dyscrasia compared to MGUS.

Signs/symptoms: Asymptomatic. Often more symptoms compared to MGUS i.e. anaemia, neuropathy or lethargy.

FBC/Blood film: Often nothing, maybe rouleaux. As disease progresses anaemia may develop, or plasma cells seen.

Diagnosis:

- PP > 30 g/l and/or
- 10–60% BM plasma cells
- No end organ damage or CRAB criteria.

Cytogenetics/molecular: t(4;14), 1q amplification or 17p deletion associated with higher chance of transformation to MM.

Subtypes: As above for MGUS.

Staging: Plasma cell % > 20, PP > 20 g/L or SFLC ratio > 20 = significant risk factor. 50% transform to MM in 5 years. Use of MRI, PET-CT or CT for bony lesion assessment.

Tx at diagnosis? No, though if very high risk and on cusp of diagnosis refer to specialist centre for consideration and closer monitoring.

Other important work up: As above for MGUS.

Emergency scenarios: Transformation to MM, amyloidosis, lymphoplasmacytoid malignancies or plasma cell leukaemia.

First line tx options: Regular monitoring under haematology not primary care of PP, SFLC and CRAB criteria every 1–3 months.

Prognosis: Risk of progression to MM: *Low*: 7–10 years. *Intermediate*: 5–6 years. *High*: 1–2 years.

Transplant: Not unless transformed to MM then consider auto in first PR or better in those eligible.

Supportive care: Neuropathy management, analgesia for bone pain, antiviral if on treatment, bone protection.

Guidelines:

https://www.kingshealthpartners.org/assets/000/003/349/Pan_London_Plasma_Cell_Guidelines_Jan_2020_original.pdf

Multiple Myeloma

Introduction: Clonal plasma cell dyscrasia characterised by hypercalcaemia, renal dysfunction, anaemia and bone pain.

Epidemiology: Second most common haematological malignancy. Incidence 5:100,000. 1% of all cancers. Male predominance. Median age over 60.

Signs/symptoms: CRAB criteria, raised total protein, hyperviscosity symptoms, pathological fractures, raised SFLC, lethargy.

FBC/Blood film: Rouleaux, anaemia, background staining increased, plasma cells present occasionally.

Diagnosis:

- Plasma cell % in BMAT > 10%.
- PP 30 g/L or more.
- CRAB criteria end organ damage as noted below.

Corrected calcium: > 2.75 or 0.25 mmol/L above baseline.

Renal: CrCl < 40 ml/minute or creatinine > 177.

Anaemia: < 100 g/L or drop of 20 g/L.

Bone lesions: 1 or more on imaging of 5 mm or more.

If CRAB criteria not met can treat based on IWMG SLIMCRAB criteria below.

SFLC ratio: ≥ 100.

Imaging: More than 1 lesion on MRI of ≥ 5 mm.

Marrow: Plasma cell percentage ≥ 60%.

Flow panel: Pos: CD38, 138, 56 and 117. **Variable:** CD20, 43, 45, 79a, IgM. **Neg:** CD19, T-cell markers.

Bone marrow: Plasma cell infiltrate, multinucleated or with immunoglobulin in cytoplasm (Russel bodies) or nucleus (Dutcher bodies).

Cytogenetics:

Intermediate risk: 1 of t(4;14), t(14;16), t(14;20), 17p-, 1q+, 1p- and B2M < 5.5.

High: Intermediate and B2M > 5.5.

Ultra-high: 2 or more from intermediate, plasma cell leukaemia or high-risk gene expression profile.

Standard: Everything else.

Molecular: *NRAS/KRAS* mutations in 40%. *BRAF* mutation in 5%. *TP53* less common but poor prognosis.

Staging: International staging system (ISS) uses B2M and albumin for median OS. Revised-ISS incorporates cytogenetics as well.

Tx at diagnosis? Yes, unless very frail or patient choice.

Other important work up: PP, SFLC, urine Bence-Jones protein, renal referral if needed, BNP, B2M, albumin, urine PCR and ACR.

Imaging: MRI as preference as per NICE but PET-CT recommended by IMWG. *Read the BSH guideline on imaging choices.*

First line tx options: Transplant ineligible vs transplant eligible. Goal is to induce deep remission, consolidate and maintain. In an ever-developing era of myeloma treatments it is important to consider eligibility and access to clinical trials or compassionate use schemes.

Transplant eligible: Dara-VTD is NICE recommended, as induction and consolidation of untreated transplant eligible adults followed by lenalidomide maintenance.

Older patients consider VTD/VCD 4–6 cycles aiming for PR or better → HDM Autograft → Lenalidomide maintenance. Daratumumab maintenance not NICE approved yet but improves PFS. If ultra-high risk, consider VTD-PACE induction with a consideration of tandem HDM autograft provided enough stem cells.

Transplant ineligible: DRD now first line. Consider Rd or Vd. If frail, consider MP or CTD. Also consider lenalidomide maintenance.

Second line: Consider clinical trial at diagnosis but especially at each relapse.

Transplant eligible: Carfilzomib if lenalidomide refractory, DVD if no daratumumab first line, Rd if not used. 2nd HDM autograft or allograft.

Transplant ineligible: DVD, CRD or Rd if not refractory or not used in first line.

Third line: IRD, velcade-panobinostat if sensitive to PI. Rd if PI refractory and not had an Imid before.

Fourth line: Daratumumab monotherapy, IsaPomDex, PomDex, velcade-panobinostat, bendamustine. CAR-T-cell therapy or other therapies like selinexor, belantamab (BCMA target) or teclistamab (bispecific) are now licensed.

Prognosis: Based on risk stratification but newer data suggesting 10-year OS around 30–35%.

Transplant: If eligible melphalan autograft in first PR or better. If high risk or relapse early post autograft, then consider a tandem autograft. Allograft considered in ultra-high risk, plasma cell leukaemia or young fit patients with relapsed refractory disease.

Response criteria: IWMG response criteria assess PP, BJP, imaging, plasma cell percentage. and SFLC.

CR: No PP, bony lesions gone or < 5% plasma cells in BM.

Stringent CR: As for CR with normal SFLC and flow -ve for plasma cells.

VGPR: > 90% reduction in PP and urine BJP < 100 mg/day.

PR: > 50% reduction in PP, plasma cells, SFLC ratio or > 90% BJP.

Important side effects of tx: Anticoagulation on lenalidomide or pomalidomide, peripheral neuropathy on velcade, osteonecrosis of jaw with zoledronic acid.

Other consideration: Late side effects i.e., other cancers or severe infections.

Supportive care: Renal input, bone protection, antiviral, fungal and bacterial prophylaxis if heavy treatment, PCP prophylaxis, hypercalcaemia management, analgesia for bone pain.

Emergency scenarios:
Malignant spinal cord compression: High dose steroids and oncology for radiotherapy. Neurosurgical involvement.
Hyperviscosity: Plasmapheresis required. Avoid blood transfusion and consider thromboprophylaxis risk.
Trials of note: Myeloma IX: Use of cytogenetics for risk stratification with B2M and albumin. CASSIOPEIA: Use of D-VTD.
Guidelines:
https://onlinelibrary.wiley.com/doi/10.1111/bjh.17410
https://www.kingshealthpartners.org/assets/000/003/349/Pan_London_Plasma_Cell_Guidelines_Jan_2020_original.pdf
https://onlinelibrary.wiley.com/doi/full/10.1111/bjh.14827

ISS staging.

Stage	Criteria
1	B2M < 3.5 mg/L and albumin > 35 g/L
2	Not meeting criteria for 1 or 3
3	B2M ≥ 5.5 mg/L

R-ISS staging.

Risk group	Criteria
1	ISS stage 1, no high-risk cytogenetic lesion and LDH within normal limits
2	Not meeting criteria for group 1 or 3
3	ISS stage 3 with high-risk cytogenetic lesion or elevated LDH

Plasma Cell Leukaemia

Introduction: Aggressive form of MM with plasma cells present in abundance in the peripheral blood.

Epidemiology: Rare but occurs in 2–4% of MM patients. Can be transformed from MM or de novo.

Signs/symptoms: MM symptoms plus B-symptoms, symptoms of cytopaenias such as infections or bleeding.

FBC/Blood film: Plasma cells present in the peripheral blood +/- cytopaenias.

Diagnosis: 20% plasma cells in the peripheral blood or > 2×10^9/L total plasma cells in the peripheral blood.

Flow panel: As for MM above.

Bone marrow: Plasma cell > 20% with maturation arrest. Plasma cells may be large with nucleoli and multinucleated forms.

Cytogenetics/Molecular: As above for MM.

Staging: Staged as ultra-high risk as per ISS or R-ISS.

Tx at diagnosis? Yes treatment as soon as possible to optimise chances of CR.

Other important work up: PP, SFLC, urine Bence-Jones protein, renal panel and referral if needed, BNP, B2M, albumin, imaging, HLA typing early, fertility, virology, G6PD.

First line tx options: VTD-PACE with auto or allo if fit and donor.

Second/third line: Trial, also consider this at diagnosis. MM therapy algorithm. Targeted therapy i.e., Daratumumab if CD38+.

Prognosis: Very poor outcomes without transplant. 6–12 months OS. Transplant extends to 2–3 years though relapse risk remains high.

Transplant: Auto consolidation in PR1 or better and consider tandem or allo if fit enough and appropriate donor.

Important side effects of tx: As above for MM.

Other consideration: Donor work up early and TLS prophylaxis.

Supportive care: As for MM but TLS prophylaxis. Consider antifungal prophylaxis more so than MM.

Guidelines:
https://www.kingshealthpartners.org/assets/000/003/349/Pan_London_Plasma_Cell_Guidelines_Jan_2020_original.pdf

Solitary Plasmacytoma of Bone (SPB) and Extramedullary Plasmacytoma (EP)

Introduction: Tumour of plasma cells presenting as solitary bony lesion or accumulation in soft tissue.

Epidemiology: 80% affect head and neck in EP. Median age of onset 60. Male sex predominance. Very rare.

Signs/symptoms: Swelling, mass, bone pain, CRAB criteria symptoms, commonly present in patients with underlying MM.

FBC/Blood film: Anaemia may be seen. Otherwise not much. 75% have PP. 50% go on to develop MM.

Diagnosis:

SBP:
- Single bony lytic lesion with plasma cells on biopsy.
- BMAT plasma cells < 10%.
- No MM defining events.

EP: As above for SBP but biopsy from soft tissue mass.

Flow panel: As above for MM.

Bone marrow: Perform to rule out MM.

Molecular/cytogenetics: As for myeloma though does not change treatment generally.

Staging: PET-CT in EP and MRI in SPB.

Tx at diagnosis? Yes.

Other important work up: As above for MM.

First line tx options: Radiotherapy and clinical oncology referral. Consider trial. If large disease, consider first line myeloma therapy. In EP if no history of MM may be related to MZL. Treat with radiotherapy +/- treatment protocol for MZL if confirmed.

Second/third line: Trial, MM chemotherapy, consider transplant.

Prognosis: Depends if underlying MM and disease site and size. Most respond in some form to radiotherapy but few studies to give statistics.

Transplant: In resistant or refractory disease consider. If underlying MM consider auto in CR1.

Supportive care: As above for MM. Bone protection. Yearly surveillance scans. Analgesia. Steroids if spinal cord compression.

Guidelines:

https://www.kingshealthpartners.org/assets/000/003/349/Pan_London_Plasma_Cell_Guidelines_Jan_2020_original.pdf

POEMS

Introduction: Paraneoplastic syndrome associated with underlying MM, MGUS or Castleman disease affecting any organ.

Incidence: Very rare, no sex predominance, can affect any age but predominantly middle age or older.

Signs/symptoms: Polyradiculopathy, organomegaly, papilloedema, sclerotic bone lesions, endocrinopathy, skin changes.

Diagnosis: Based on mandatory criteria of polyradiculopathy and plasma cell disorder with 1 major and 1 minor criteria:

- <u>Major</u>: Castleman disease, sclerotic bone lesions or elevated VEGF.
- <u>Minor</u>: Organomegaly, oedema, endocrinopathy, skin change, papilloedema and thrombocytosis.

Flow panel: If MM clone then markers for plasma cell clone.

Bone marrow: Useful for guiding treatment if plasma cell neoplasm.

Tx at diagnosis? If plasma cell clone or > 3 bony lesions yes. If not, can monitor closely.

Other important work up: Hormone panels, CT for organomegaly, imaging for bone lesions, lung function, VEGF levels for monitoring treatment responses and disease activity.

First line tx options: Consider radiotherapy if only 1 bony site. Systemic therapy if plasma cell clone or multiple lesions. Melphalan + Dexamethasone or imid based therapy. Consider velcade triple therapy if well and no contraindication i.e., neuropathy.

Second/third line: Clinical trials. Imid based therapy if not tried previously.

Prognosis: 80% have haematological response to melphalan. Those who survive and have auto generally do well.

Transplant: Autograft with high dose melphalan in CR1 in those fit who have underlying plasma cell clone.

Supportive care: Specialist input for organ system affected, bone protection, antibacterial/viral agents as per MM treatment.

Guidelines:
https://www.kingshealthpartners.org/assets/000/003/349/Pan_London_Plasma_Cell_Guidelines_Jan_2020_original.pdf

AL Amyloidosis

Introduction: Systemic disorder associated with plasma cell clone leading to profound amyloid deposition throughout the body commonly affecting the kidneys, heart and GI tract.

Epidemiology: Rare, 1:100,000 incidence, median age of onset 50–70. No sex predominance.

Signs/symptoms: Nephrotic syndrome, cardiomyopathy, peripheral neuropathy, hepatomegaly, autonomic neuropathy, GI symptoms, macroglossia, orbital ecchymosis, thrombosis. Any organ can be involved.

Diagnosis: Presence of amyloid deposition in tissue diagnosed by Congo-Red stain with apple green birefringence under polarised light and plasma cell infiltrate. Multiple tissue biopsies may be needed but not recommended. SAP scan showing amyloid deposition.

Flow panel: +ve markers for plasma cell dyscrasia as above.

Bone marrow: Recommended at diagnosis for estimate of plasma cell infiltrate, Congo-Red staining +ve and cytogenetics.

Cytogenetics/Molecular: As for MM above though treatment largely the same irrespective.

Staging: Troponin T > 0.003 ng/ml and/or NT pro-BNP > 335 pg/ml. If BNP > 8500 pg/ml = worst prognosis.

Tx at diagnosis? Yes, and consider clinical trial at diagnosis.

Other important work up: As for MM and Nt-Pro-BNP, troponin, nerve conduction if neuropathy and anti-GAD antibodies, cardiac MRI, SAP scan, endoscopy for GI symptoms, renal referral, analysis of amyloid fibril subtype, SFLC measurement in response, urine PCR and ACR. Refer all to National Amyloid Centre.

First line tx options: Typically, myeloma style treatment i.e., VRD or VTD. Melphalan and dexamethasone in pulses.

Second/third line: Trial. Lenalidomide or pomalidomide. Autograft.

Prognosis: Overall survival based on stage.

Stage 1: 8 years.

Stage 2: 3–4 years.

Stage 3/4: 6–12 months.

Response: Monitoring SFLC after each cycle. Measurement of PP. Response criteria based on organ affected and biochemical marker improvement i.e., for cardiac amyloidosis a drop in NT-Pro-BNP and improved NHYA classification.

Transplant: Consider in CR1 if high risk. In relapse or refractory disease. Higher risk in those with cardiac amyloid, GI bleeding, advanced renal disease or pleural involvement. Goal is to achieve VGPR or better with transplant.

Important side effects of tx: Caution with thalidomide in cardiac disease due to arrythmias.

Supportive care: Diuresis, anticoagulation if on Imid, doxycycline shown to improve outcomes when combined with chemotherapy as interferes with amyloid fibril formation, antibiotic and antiviral prophylaxis, loop device for arrhythmia monitoring.
Guidelines:
https://rmpartners.nhs.uk/wp-content/uploads/2020/01/Pan-London-Plasma-Cell-Guidelines-Jan-2020.pdf
https://onlinelibrary.wiley.com/doi/full/10.1111/bjh.13156
https://onlinelibrary.wiley.com/doi/full/10.1111/bjh.13155

Myelodysplastic and Bone Marrow Failure Syndromes

Myelodysplastic Syndrome

Introduction: Group of clonal haematopoietic stem cell disorders encompassed by ineffective haematopoiesis with an array of underlying cytogenetic abnormalities influencing the spectrum of disease severity. Disease phenotype can range from active monitoring as an outpatient to transformation to AML.

Epidemiology: Rises with age. 5:100,000 incidence normally in all age groups but 35:100,000 in 70–80-year-olds.

Signs/symptoms: Asymptomatic in many, symptoms of cytopaenias such as anaemia, bleeding or infections. B-symptoms can occur such as fevers or splenomegaly.

FBC/Blood film: Macrocytosis on FBC with cytopaenias. Film may show pseudo-Pelger cells, hypo-granulated neutrophils, blasts, internuclear bridging of white cells, basophilic stippling of red cells, giant platelets, hypolobated white cells.

Diagnosis: Based on WHO criteria for each subdivision of MDS, see below. For lineage to be dysplastic needs to be ≥ 10% of cells.

Flow panel: Useful for assessing myeloid blast presence and percentage.

Bone marrow: Examination of > 500 cells to assess dysplasia.

Dyserythropoiesis: Internuclear bridging, karyorrhexis, multinuclearity, megaloblastic change.

Dysmyelopoiesis: Small or large forms, hyper/hyposegmentation, hypogranularity, Döhle bodies, blasts +/- Auer rods.

Dysmegakaropoiesis: Micromegakaryocytes, nuclear hypolobation, multinucleation.

Cytogenetics: Most common are abnormalities of chromosomes 5, 7, 11, 13, 17.

Molecular: 50–70% have 1 mutation. Commonest include: *SF3B, TET2, RUNX1, ASXL1, SRSF2, TP53, NRAS/KRAS, DNMT3A*.

Staging:

IPSS: Blasts, karyotype and cytopaenias.

IPSS-R: Cytogenetics, blasts, Hb, platelets, neutrophil count.

Both used for median OS.

IPSS-Mol: As above including molecular abnormalities.

Tx at diagnosis? Depends on risk category, patient frailty and type of MDS.

Other important work up: Virology, PP, HLA typing, EPO, haematinics, iron panel, haptoglobins, parvovirus, reticulocytes, DAT, LDH.

First line tx options:

Low/intermediate risk: Active monitoring, EPO, GCSF, ATG/ciclosporin in hypocellular, lenalidomide in del 5q.

Intermediate/high: Azacitadine or decitabine if not transplant eligible in combination with lenalidomide or venetoclax if funded.

If transplant eligible and high-risk, goal is allograft after induction chemotherapy.

Second/third line: Trial, lenalidomide or venetoclax if not tried before. If molecular mutations, consider targeted therapy.

Prognosis: Depends on risk stratification.

Low risk: OS 6–10 years.

High risk: OS 1-year without allo.

Transplant: Allo in CR1 in high risk who are suitable and have appropriate donor. No role for auto.

Important side effects of tx: Iron chelation to consider from transfusion, transfusion reactions, antibody formation form transfusion, azacitadine side effects as per AML above.

Supportive care: Transfusion support, antibiotics, antivirals, PCP prophylaxis. Higher chance of morbidity and mortality from infection rather than transformation so good patient education and support network, often older patients with co-morbidities so MDT approach.

Guidelines:

https://rmpartners.nhs.uk/wp-content/uploads/2020/01/Pan-London-MDS-Guideline-Jan-2020.pdf

https://onlinelibrary.wiley.com/doi/10.1111/bjh.17612

MDS IPSS

Criteria	Score of 0	Score of 0.5	Score of 1	Score of 1.5	Score of 2
BM Blast %	< 5	5–10	-	10–19	≥ 20
Cytopaenias	0–1	≥ 2	-	-	-
Karyotype	Good: Normal, loss of Y, deletion 5q or 20q	Intermediate: all others	Poor: Complex karyotype or abnormalities of 7	-	-

Total score	Risk
0	Low
0.5–1	Intermediate 1
1.5–2	Intermediate 2
> 2	High

MDS cytogenetic mutations and the risk groups they fall into.

Risk group	Cytogenetic lesion
Very good	Deletion 11q or loss of Y chromosome
Good	No cytogenetic lesion or single deletion 5q, 12p, 20q. Double deletion 5q
Intermediate	Single deletion 7q, inversion 7q or gain of 8 or 19. Double deletion or gain of any other cytogenetic mutation
Poor	Single deletion of 7 or 3q abnormalities. Double abnormalities in 7 or 7q. Complex karyotype with 3 mutations
Very poor	Complex karyotype with greater than 3 mutations

MDS R-IPSS. Uses more in-depth cytogenetics as well as individual cytopaenias.

Criteria	Score of 0	Score of 0.5	Score of 1	Score of 1.5	Score of 2	Score of 3	Score of 4
Blast %	≤ 2	-	2.1–4.9	-	5–10	≥ 10	
Cytogenetic risk group	Very good	-	Good	-	Intermediate	Poor	Very poor
Haemoglobin g/L	≥ 100	-	80–99	< 80	-	-	-
Platelets × 10⁹/L	≥ 100	50–99	< 50	-	-	-	-
Neutrophil count × 10⁹/L	≥ 0.8	< 0.8	-	-	-	-	-

Total score	Risk
≤ 1.5	Very low
1.6–3	Low
3.1–4.5	Intermediate 1
4.6-6	Intermediate 2
> 6	High

MDS 2022 WHO classification.

MDS subtype	Blast % in BM and PB	Cytogenetic	Molecular
MDS with low blasts and isolated *SF3B1*	< 5% BM and < 2% PB	Any except 3q, 5q, 7q deletions or complex karyotype	*SF3B1* mutation ≥ 10% VAF without *TP53* or *RUNX1* mutation
MDS with low blasts and isolated del(5q)	< 5% BM and < 2% PB	Deletion 5q. An additional cytogenetic abnormality can occur also except deletion 7 or 7q	Any allowed except multi hit mutations of *TP53*
MDS with multi-hit *TP53* mutations	0–19% in both	17p deletions or mutations. Often complex karyotype	Multi-hit *TP53* mutations or *TP53* mutation with > 10% VAF and complex karyotype
MDS post-cytotoxic chemotherapy	Variable	Not meeting other criteria and history of previous systemic high-dose chemotherapy	Variable
MDS with low blasts	< 5% BM and < 2% PB	Any except those fulfilling above criteria	Any except those fulfilling above criteria
MDS with increased blasts 1	5–9% BM and 2–4% PB	Any except those fulfilling above criteria	Any except those fulfilling above criteria
MDS with increased blasts 2	10–19% BM and 5–19% PB. Or Auer rods	Any except those fulfilling above criteria	Any except those fulfilling above criteria
Hypoplastic MDS	< 5% and < 2% and hypocellular BM	Variable, often none. Not meeting any criteria above	Variable, often none. Not meeting any criteria above
MDS with fibrosis	5–19% BM and 2–19% PB. Fibrotic BM	Any except those fulfilling above criteria	Any except those fulfilling above criteria
MDS unclassifiable	< 5% BM and < 2% PB	Not meeting any criteria above	Not meeting any criteria above

CHIP, CCUS and ICUS

Introduction: Syndromes of clonal haematopoiesis with associated MDS mutation without clinical features of MDS.

Epidemiology: Increasing incidence with age. Found in > 10% of people over the age of 70.

Signs/symptoms: Often none, mild anaemia or cytopenia may trigger investigation.

Diagnosis: Presence of either clonal haematopoiesis, cytopaenias, MDS related molecular mutations not meeting MDS criteria.

Flow panel: Often not useful but may show small presence of myeloid blasts but not significant enough to meet MDS criteria.

Bone marrow: May reflect dysplasia in lineage with cytopaenias but not significant enough to diagnose MDS.

Cytogenetics/Molecular: Commonly mutated *DNMT3A, TET2, ASXL1, IDH2* and *TP53*. Commonly < 10% allelic frequency.

Subtypes:

CHIP: Somatic mutations associated with MDS or myeloid malignancy in PB or BM without haematological disorder.

ICUS: 1 or more unexplained cytopaenias not diagnostic of MDS or haematological disorder.

CCUS: 1 or more unexplained cytopaenias with clonal haematopoiesis not diagnostic of MDS or haematological disorder.

Tx at diagnosis? No, but regular monitoring suggested.

Other important work up: Rule out haematological malignancy or other marrow infiltrate, USS for splenomegaly, virology, drug causes for cytopaenias, autoimmune screen, haematinics.

First line tx options: Monitoring based on number of mutations and severity of cytopaenias.

Prognosis: CHIP < 1% per year risk of progression to haematological malignancy. ICUS 9% at 10 years. CCUS higher risk for progression.

Transplant: Not considered unless progression to high risk MDS or AML.

Supportive care: Antibiotics if infections, occasionally transfusion support if symptomatic or other co-morbidities.

Guidelines:

https://onlinelibrary.wiley.com/doi/full/10.1111/bjh.17621

Other Myelodysplastic Syndromes

A brief overview. These have recently been reclassified by the international consensus classification from the WHO 2017 guidance. Their reclassification now has JMML falling under paediatrics and germline associated disorders. Atypical CML, CMML and MDS/MPN NOS remain with the addition of CMUS, MDS/MPN-T-SF3B1, MDS/MPN with isolated (17q) and MDS/MPN-RS-T, NOS.

Atypical CML

Introduction: Rare, BCR-ABL-1 -ve CML with evidence of dysplasia predominantly affecting neutrophils.
Diagnosis:
- WCC > 13×10^9/L,
- Ph chromosome or *PDGFRA/B* -ve,
- Neutrophil precursors, granulopoiesis, dysplasia and cytopaenias
- No CML/CMML criteria.
- Absence of monocytosis or eosinophilia, hypergranular bone marrow.

MDS/MPN NOS

Introduction: Features of MDS and MPN that do not fulfil other criteria such as CMML etc.
Diagnosis:
- MDS features.
- No AML criteria.
- MPN diagnostic criteria met.
- No CML or molecular mutations associated with other disorder i.e., *PDGFRA*.
- Blasts < 20%.

Clonal Monocytosis of Undetermined Significance

Introduction: Persistent monocytosis without dysplasia or blasts but associated myeloid neoplastic mutation not meeting other MDS/MPN or CML criteria.
Diagnosis:
- Monocytosis $\geq 0.5 \times 10^9$/L and 10% of WCC.
- No dysplasia, cytopaenias or other reactive cause.
- Not meeting the criteria for CML or other MPN.
- Associated myeloid neoplastic mutation.

MDS/MPN with Thrombocytosis and *SF3B1* Mutation

Introduction: Thrombocytosis with associated dysplasia and cytopaenias and *SF3B1* mutation not meeting the criteria of other MDS/MPN syndromes.

Diagnosis:
- Thrombocytosis $\geq 450 \times 10^9$/L.
- Anaemia.
- Blasts < 1 % in PB and < 5% in BM.
- *SF3B1* mutation with VAF > 10%.
- No other associated mutations fitting with CML or other myeloid neoplasm.
- No history of MDS or MPN.
- No chemotherapy or medications which would cause MDS/MPN BM appearance.

MDS/MPN with Isolated Isochrome (17q)

Introduction: MDS/MPN crossover associated with isolated isochrome 17q or in combination with another molecular mutation except deletion 7 or 7q.

Diagnosis:
- WCC > 13×10^9/L.
- Fulfils MDS/MPN NOS criteria.
- Cytopaenias.
- Blasts < 20% in PB or BM.
- Hypolobated neutrophils or pseudo-Pelger cells morphologically.
- Isolated isochrome 17q mutation.
- Absence of CML or MPN mutations.
- No recent chemotherapy which would cause MDS/MPN BM appearance.

MDS/MPN with Ring Sideroblasts, Thrombocytosis NOS

Introduction: Like MDS/MPN NOS but thrombocytosis, ring sideroblasts excess, absence of *SF3B1* mutation and lower blast threshold.

Diagnosis:
- Thrombocytosis $\geq 450 \times 10^9$/L.
- Anaemia.
- Erythroid dysplasia with ring sideroblasts in BM $\geq 15\%$.
- Clonal molecular or cytogenetic mutations.
- Blast < 1 % in PB and 5% in BM.
- Absence of *SF3B1* mutation or other MDS/MPN or CML defining mutations.
- No recent chemotherapy which would cause MDS/MPN BM appearance.

Chronic Myelomonocytic Leukaemia: See below

Chronic Myelomonocytic Leukaemia

Introduction: Dysplastic condition with different phases, that is associated with persistent monocytosis, dysplasia and presence of blasts.

Epidemiology: 1:10,000. Slight male predominance and median age of onset 65–75.

Signs/symptoms: High WCC, cytopaenias, splenomegaly, B-symptoms, fatigue, bleeding, infections.

FBC/Blood film: Monocytosis, anaemia or other cytopaenias, dysplastic features, myeloid blasts, abnormal monocytes, occasionally eosinophilia or basophilia.

Diagnosis:

- PB monocytosis $> 0.5 \times 10^9$/L without reactive cause for 3 months.
- Absence of Ph chromosome or other MPN defining mutation.
- $< 20\%$ blasts in PB or BM.
- Absence of *PDGFRA/B* rearrangements or other eosinophilia defining gene rearrangement.
- Supporting criteria though not diagnostic: 1. Dysplasia in ≥ 1 myeloid line. 2. Acquired clonal or cytogenetic abnormality. 3. Abnormal PB monocyte subsets.

Flow panel: Pos: CD13, 14, 33, 64, 68. **Variable:** CD33 associated with AML transformation. CD14 reflects monocyte immaturity. CD2 and 56 occasionally +ve also. **Neg:** T-cell markers and B-cell markers. CD13, 15, 36, HLA-DR.

Bone marrow: Granulocyte dysplasia and proliferation, hypercellular marrow, increased monocytes, ring sideroblasts, megaloblastic changes, micro-megakaryocytes or hypolobated forms.

Cytogenetics: 20–40% of cases. -7, +8 and 12p abnormalities.

Good risk: Normal or loss of Y.

Intermediate risk: Other abnormalities not in good or poor risk.

Poor risk: Gain of 8, abnormalities affecting 7 or complex karyotype with more than 3 abnormalities.

Molecular: Vast array of mutations including *SF3B1, RUNX1 CBL, SRSF2, TET2, ASXL1, NRAS, EZH2*.

Staging: Scoring is CPSS or Dusseldorf scoring systems for prognosis.

CPSS: Based on subtype, white cell count, cytogenetics and transfusion dependence.

Dusseldorf scoring system: Blast count, haemoglobin, LDH and platelets.

CMML-0: Blasts $< 2\%$ PB and $< 5\%$ BM.

CMML-1: Blasts $< 5\%$ Pb and 10% BM.

CMML-2: Blasts $< 19\%$ in PB or BM.

Proliferative: WCC $\geq 13 \times 10^9$/L.

Dysplastic: WCC $< 13 \times 10^9$/L.

Tx at diagnosis? Depends on stage. If CMML-1 or less, then can have active monitoring.

Other important work up: Fertility counselling, virology and atypical infections, USS for splenomegaly, HLA typing.

First line tx options: Hydroxycarbamide to control counts if no excess of blasts. Azacitadine for CMML-2. AML based chemotherapy such as DA for CMML-2 with high count or those who have transformed followed by allograft.

Second/third line: Trial or AML chemotherapy if refractory or progressive disease. Other hypomethylating agent i.e., decitabine.

Prognosis: Progression to AML in 15–30%. OS 2–4 years.

Transplant: Allograft in those suitable and in high-risk disease or CMML-2 or transformation to AML.

Important side effects of tx: As above for AML treatments and hydroxycarbamide.

Other consideration: Symptomatic splenomegaly and transfusion support. Infection risk and functional hyposplenism.

Supportive care: Antibiotics, antiviral prophylaxis, vaccinations, PCP prophylaxis, transfusion support.

Guidelines:
https://rmpartners.nhs.uk/wp-content/uploads/2020/01/Pan-London-MDS-Guideline-Jan-2020.pdf

Aplastic Anaemia

Introduction: Bone marrow failure syndrome with varying severity. It can be inherited or acquired with underlying causes including drugs, infection, PNH, Fanconi's anaemia or other rare inherited conditions. Most cases idiopathic.

Epidemiology: Rare. Incidence of 2.5:1,000,000. Bimodal peak of TYA and > 60-years-old.

Signs/symptoms: Shortness of breath, bleeding, infection, lethargy, petechiae, sepsis and other symptoms of pancytopaenia.

FBC/Blood film: Depending on severity can be mild cytopaenias or severe pancytopaenia.

Diagnosis: Absence of leukaemia or fibrosis and 2 of below:
- Hb < 100 g/L.
- Platelet < 50 × 10⁹/L.
- Neutrophils < 1.5 × 10⁹/L.

Flow panel: Unless PNH clone present flow is of little use. PNH clone +ve for GPI-anchored proteins. CD14, 16, 24. FLAER for CD55 and CD59. Small PNH clone seen in 50% of AA patients. Test regularly to assess for evolving clone which was undetectable previously.

Bone marrow: Hypocellular marrow without fibrosis or infiltrate.

Cytogenetics: Abnormalities of 5, 7, 8, 13 commonly.

Molecular: Heterogenous. GATA2 mutation in Emberger syndrome. SBDS mutation in SDS. Other myeloid panel mutations seen too.

Staging:

Camitta criteria:

Severe: Marrow < 25% cellularity and 2 of; neutrophils < 0.5 × 10⁹/L, platelets < 20 × 10⁹/L and reticulocytes < 20 × 10⁹/L.

Very Severe: As above but neutrophils < 0.2 × 10⁹/L.

Non-severe: Not fulfilling severe or very severe criteria.

Tx at diagnosis? Not always, supportive care if non-severe. If underlying disorder treat disorder first.

Other important work up: Retics, HbF, chromosomal breakage for FA, flow for GPI anchorage proteins, virology including parvovirus, LFTs, haematinics, autoimmune screen, examination for clinical signs of telomere shortening.

First line tx options: Based on age of patient.

Age ≤ 35: Sibling donor Allograft. No donor Haplo/MUD or Horse ATG with CSA.

Age 35–50: As above or trial of horse ATG and CSA first. No response after 3–6 months then proceed to HLA/MUD or haplo allograft.

Age > 50: Horse ATG and CSA first. Then follow 35–50 algorithm if no response.

Second/third line: Persistent cytopaenias classifies disease as refractory. If suitable donor, then proceed to allograft. If no donor another trial or ATG and CSA while donor work up. Alemtuzumab, MMF, androgens or eltrombopag. Trial.

Prognosis: Good ATG response if young less severe disease, retics $> 25 \times 10^9$/L, lymphocytes $> 1 \times 10^9$/L, trisomy 8 or del(13q).

Response: <u>Severe</u>:

None: Still fulfil criteria of AA at diagnosis.

Partial: Transfusion independent.

Complete: Platelets $< 150 \times 10^9$/L, neutrophils $> 1.5 \times 10^9$/L and Hb normal.

<u>In non-severe AA</u>:

None: Worse counts.

Partial: As above + doubling of 1 or more cell line or baseline Hb increase > 30 g/L, neutrophils $> 0.5 \times 10^9$/L and platelets $> 20 \times 10^9$/L.

Complete: As above for severe.

Transplant: Yes, allograft ideally from sibling or haplo. MUD if no appropriate donors. Autograft not used.

Important side effects of tx: ATG reactions with fever and rigors. Iron loading based on transfusion history.

Other consideration: Regular red cell antibody screening. Irradiated products if ATG or allo planned. Rh and Kell phenotyped blood if possible. PCP not required. Consider fungal prophylaxis if severe prolonged neutropaenia. Consider iron chelation.

Supportive care: Regular transfusion support, GCSF, prophylactic antibiotics and antivirals. Iron chelation.

Guidelines:

https://onlinelibrary.wiley.com/doi/full/10.1111/bjh.13853

Transfusion

This chapter has been the toughest to write in terms of a structure for an essay as there are many different types of topics to cover but I have largely followed the same structure for each section, except for lab principles. The beginner and intermediate transfusion courses are ESSENTIAL for deep understanding of transfusion principles and the exam. The one thing I would say about transfusion is pick carefully when you do the 3-week transfusion course. Doing it too early before the exam leaves you open to having to learn it all again on your own. Leaving it too late may mean you won't have time to build up your knowledge around the subjects you have learned. The majority of the information is taken from the BSH guidelines, good practice papers or JPAC and NHSBT guidance.

Blood Products

Red Cells

Introduction: The transfusion of packed red cells as a "unit" typically around 400–500 ml in volume, is used to treat anaemia due to various causes when other treatments or managements are not suitable. "The safest transfusion is the one that doesn't need to happen".

Epidemiology: New donations in 2019/20 lowest since 2016, with 130,000.

Donation steps:
1. Locate suitable ACF vein.
2. Clean arm with antiseptic solution and wait to dry.
3. Check whole blood pack for date and time as well as inspect for damage of pack.
4. Insert needle.
5. 30 ml divert for serology and group testing.
6. Fill to desired bag volume, mean 470 ml in 63 ml CPD anticoagulant bag.
7. Monitor throughout.
8. Remove needle and provide aftercare.

Production: Whole blood is leucodepleted via filtration to reduced incidence of febrile reaction, antibody formation or vCJD infection. $< 1 \times 10^6$/L WCC left. Centrifuged to separate plasma, platelets and RBC. Bag squeezed to separate the 3 components into individual bags.

Donor selection: Age 17–65, 50–158 kg, 3–4 months between donations, passed donor selection questionnaire, Hb > 125/135 g/L for women and men.

Cannot donate if: High risk for prion exposure as per JPAC, BBV or high risk of BBV based on questionnaire, not meeting donor selection guidance, previous malignancy, clinical indication not too, solid organ transplant, use of IV drugs, previous stem cell transplant. May be deferred based on sexual history and PREP or PEP use in last 3 months.

Groups: <u>Most to least common ABO/Rh grouping</u>: O+, A+, O-, A-, B+, B-, AB+, AB-. Other groups discussed later.

Screened for:

<u>Routinely</u>: Anti-HIV 1 and 2 antibody and HIV NAT, HBsAg, anti-HCV antibody and HCV NAT, anti-HTLV-1 and 2 antibody, syphilis antibodies.

<u>Additional</u>: Malaria, CMV, West Nile and *T. Cruzi* antibodies based on travel history or those requiring CMV -ve.

Product half-life: 35 days at 4°C. Transfuse within 4 hours. Up to 60 minutes out of lab can still be returned.

Safety mechanisms: Patient education, appropriate donor selection, leucodepleted by filtration to reduce TA-GvHD, irradiation if needed.

Product requirements: Volume 220–350 ml, HCT 0.5–0.7, Hb > 40 g/L, suspended in SAG-M additive solution.

Clinical assessment: Assess for risk of TACO, TRALI or other transfusion reaction, current infection and fever monitoring, patient weight and target Hb, other considerations like oral or IV iron needed or EPO.

Ask yourself: Can the transfusion wait? Is it clinically urgent? Are there other means to raise Hb? Is there associated risk of transfusions? Is this patient suitable for transfusion?

Targets (g/L): Be restrictive!

Surgery: > 70 or 80 if symptomatic or bleeding.

ITU: *Early sepsis:* > 90. *Late sepsis:* > 70. *Ischaemia:* >90. *SAH:* > 80. *ACS:* > 80. *Angina:* > 70. *Haemodynamically unstable:* > 90. *Stable in ITU:* > 70.

Healthy: Consider other treatments if stable and asymptomatic. Target of > 70 generally but if well and due to other cause like B12 deficiency then replace first.

Minimum grouping required: ABO and Rh grouping as well as antibody screening and above infection screening. 2 sample policy on group and save and crossmatching blood in hospital to reduce risk of WBIT.

Important side effects: Transfusion reactions either acute or delayed i.e., TACO, TRALI, etc, risk of BBV or bacterial infection, risk of alloantibody formation, allergy in IgA deficient, TA-GvHD.

Monitoring: Patient ID using 3 identifiers, documentation of transfusion details including, pre, peri and post-transfusion, communication with patients and duty of candour if mistakes or near misses happen, documented patient consent, traceability of donor in case of reaction by recipient, observations within 60 minutes pre-transfusion, 15 minutes after starting and 60 minutes after completion.

Trials to quote: TRICC: Restrictive transfusion threshold in ITU patients did not worsen outcomes and lower mortality in restrictive group.

Other considerations: Training for staff every 3 years, competency assessments by MHRA, labelling of group and save at patient bedside by the person who took the blood and should be handwritten, positive patient identification, in non-emergency transfuse 1 unit then reassess.

Guidelines:

https://onlinelibrary.wiley.com/doi/full/10.1111/tme.12481

https://www.transfusionguidelines.org/transfusion-handbook/3-providing-safe-blood/3-3-blood-products.pdf

Platelets

Introduction: The transfusion of platelets as a "pool" from 4 donors typically around 300 ml in volume, used to treat thrombocytopaenia or bleeding when other treatments or managements are not suitable. They can be pooled from multiple donor whole blood donation or single donor from apheresis.

Epidemiology: 275,000 transfusion per year. Accounts for 2/3 of transfusions in haematological malignancies.

Production: As above but the buffy coats are taken when centrifuged, which is the layer between RBC and plasma, from 4 donors and pooled. In single donor the platelets are taken directly via apheresis machine before the other blood constituents are returned to the donor via the other arm.

Donor selection: Age 17–65, 50–158 kg, 12–16 weeks between donation, passed donor selection questionnaire, Hb > 125/135 g/L for women and men.

Cannot donate if: As above.

Groups: A, B, O or AB. AB very rare. Mismatch leads to reduced platelet survival but compared to ABO mismatch for RBC this is not clinically that significant. Small chance of anti-A and B antibodies in platelets from plasma collected so give group O platelets to O recipients. Give RhD -ve platelets to RhD -ve women of childbearing age.

Screened for: As above.

Product half-life: 5 days at 20–24°C at constant agitation. Transfused over 30 minutes.

Safety mechanisms: Patient education, appropriate donor selection, irradiation if needed, leucodepletion, blood culture.

Product requirements:

Pooled: Volume 300 ml, mean platelets of 308×10^9 per unit, stored in CPD anticoagulant in plasma of another donor.

Apheresis: Volume of 199 ml from 1 donor, mean platelets of 280×10^9 per unit, stored in ACD anticoagulant.

Others: In PAS for those with severe allergy, irradiated, HLA selected or HPA 1a/5b -ve for those with antibodies.

HLA matched products require irradiation.

Clinical assessment: Assess for risk of TACO, TRALI or other transfusion reaction, current infection and fever monitoring, patient weight and target count, other considerations like TXA or other local measure to stop bleeding.

Ask yourself: Can the transfusion wait? Is it clinically urgent? Are there other means to raise platelet count? Is there associated risk of transfusions? Is this patient suitable for transfusion?

Targets (× 10⁹/L): Be restrictive!

Prophylaxis no bleeding: > 10.

Prophylaxis no bleeding and fever: > 20.

Major bleeding: > 50.

Minor bleeding: > 30.

LP: > 50.

Major surgery: > 50.

Liver biopsy: > 50.

Epidural: > 80.

ICB, life-threatening bleeding or neurosurgery: > 100.

Minimum grouping required: ABO grouping on platelets. HLA and HPA antibodies requested via NHSBT after proof of fail to increment or know antibodies. 2 sample policy on group and save, and crossmatching blood in hospital to reduce risk of WBIT.

Important side effects: As above + higher chance of bacterial infection due to storage conditions. Higher chance of TRALI in platelets from female donors who have had children.

Monitoring: As above.

Trials to quote: PATCH: Platelet transfusion after head injury with ICB worsened outcomes compared to those who did not receive.

Other considerations: Training for staff every 3 years, competency assessments by MHRA, labelling of group and save at patient bedside by the person who took the blood and should be handwritten, positive patient identification, in non-emergency transfuse 1 pool then reassess.

Guidelines:

https://onlinelibrary.wiley.com/doi/full/10.1111/bjh.14423.

https://www.transfusionguidelines.org/transfusion-handbook/3-providing-safe-blood/3-3-blood-products.pdf

Plasma Products

Introduction: The transfusion of plasma can be as FFP, cryoprecipitate or in various other derivatives such as IVIG. Plasma products are used to treat disorders primarily of fibrinogen or factor deficiency commonly in bleeding in DIC. They are also used as prophylaxis in conditions prior to procedures such as liver disease awaiting a biopsy or surgical intervention.

Production: As above + frozen immediately to preserve clotting factors. Can be donated via apheresis also.

Donor selection: As above but generally male only to reduce risk of TRALI.

Cannot donate if: As above.

Groups: ABO grouping with group matched if possible. If not, then AB or low titre A or B matched. Reserve group O plasma for group O recipients.

Screened for: As above.

Product half-life: Can be stored up to 36 months at -25°C or below, once FFP thawed in water bath can be kept at 4°C for 24 hours. Cryo used within 4 hours of thawing.

Safety mechanisms: Patient education, Appropriate donor selection, irradiation if needed, leucodepletion, blood culture and virology testing.

Product requirements:

FFP: Single donor, volume of 274 ml, factor VIII concentration > 0.7 IU/ml, suspended in CPD anticoagulant.

SD-FFP: Up to 1520 donors per batch, 200 ml volume, factor VIII concentration > 0.5 IU/ml, mean fibrinogen concentration 2.6 mg/ml, sodium citrate anticoagulant, can be stored up to 4 years if needed.

Cryo: Either as pack (1 donor) or pool (5 donors). 1 × pool mean volume 189 ml, fibrinogen mg/pack > 700, factor VIII > 350 IU.

MB-FFP: Generally imported plasma treated with Methylene blue to reduce risk of viral transmission. Preferred in paediatrics. Single donor. Reduced activity of fibrinogen and factor VIII.

Plasma derivatives:

IVIG: From large pools of donor plasma with antibodies against pathogens or for replacement therapy.

HAS: No blood antigens or clotting factors. Often used following ascitic drainage or severe hypoalbuminemia.

Fibrinogen concentrate: Licensed in congenital hypofibrinogenemia only. From large donor pools.

PCC: From large donor pools. Contains factors II, VII, IX, X. Used in warfarin and DOACS reversal.

Clinical assessment: Assess for risk of TACO, TRALI or other transfusion reaction, current infection and fever monitoring, patient weight and target count, other considerations like TXA or other local measure to stop bleeding.

Ask yourself: Can the transfusion wait? Is it clinically urgent? Are there other means to raise platelet count? Is there associated risk of transfusions? Is this patient suitable for transfusion?

Targets: Be restrictive! Used in bleeding with associated factor or fibrinogen deficiency commonly or in major haemorrhage.

Important side effects: Risk of severe allergic reactions, TRALI more likely with plasma.

Monitoring: As above.

Other considerations: As above + people born after 1996 only receive plasma from countries with low risk of vCJD. Hepatitis and TB serological tests are false +ve after administration of plasma.

Guidelines:

https://onlinelibrary.wiley.com/doi/full/10.1111/bjh.14423

https://www.transfusionguidelines.org/transfusion-handbook/3-providing-safe-blood/3-3-blood-products.pdf

Granulocytes

Introduction: The transfusion of granulocytes is becoming less frequent but is still occasionally used in life threatening sepsis and neutropaenia which is prolonged because of toxins or drugs where patients are not responding to antibiotics.

Production: As above but following separation into individual products the buffy coat is removed from plasma-red cell junction. Can also be collected via single donor apheresis. Exist as pooled buffy coat granulocytes, apheresis single donor and pooled in additive solution or plasma.

Donor selection: As above for other blood products.

Cannot donate if: As above.

Groups: ABO and Rh grouping required due to risk of red cell contamination and ABO incompatibility.

Screened for: As above.

Product half-life: Stored at 20–24°C and agitated (unless in additive solution and plasma). Use within 24 hours for single donor apheresis or midnight on the day of collection for others.

Product requirements:

Buffy coat: Mean volume per pack is 60 ml, often 10 packs used at a dose of 1×10^{10} cells/ pack. Hct: 0.45. Platelets: 70×10^9/L.

Pooled: Less red cell and plasma contamination and resuspended in plasma to reduce TRALI risk. 207 ml/pack, dose is 2 packs. 1×10^{10} cells/pack, Hct: 0.15. Platelets: 499×10^9/L.

Single donor apheresis: GCSF and steroids beforehand, 312 ml/pack, $> 1 \times 10^9$ cells/ pack.

Targets: No specific target but used in severe neutropaenia not responding to antibiotics with +ve bacterial or fungal culture.

Important side effects: Risk of acute or delayed transfusion reaction. Risk of infection due to storage conditions.

Monitoring: As above.

Other considerations: Irradiated to reduce risk of TA-GvHD in immunocompromised patient and leucodepleted.

Guidelines:

https://onlinelibrary.wiley.com/doi/full/10.1111/bjh.14423

https://www.transfusionguidelines.org/transfusion-handbook/3-providing-safe-blood/3-3-blood-products.pdf

Transfusion Alternatives

I have split them into pre-operative, peri-operative salvage techniques and pharmacological methods including adjuncts to reduce the bleeding risk. In a question like this always consider holistic approaches such as paediatric blood tubes and asking the person why they wish to refuse a transfusion and exploring their ideas, concerns, and expectations. It's also important to clarify which products people may or may not wish to receive.

Pre-deposit autologous donation (PAD)

Introduction: A donation of up to 3 units prior to surgery. Processed as per allogenic donation. Iron or EPO given to prevent anaemia.

Indications: Patient preference, rare blood types or antibodies, paediatric or surgery were significant likelihood of transfusion.

Cautions: Risk of anaemia, stored for 35 days at 4°C, risk of surgery being cancelled and donation lost, risk of extra bleeding.

Other considerations: Assess ability to donate safely, used in exceptional circumstances only in reality.

Cell salvage

Introduction: Intra or post-op cell salvage from blood loss during surgery. Automated devices which filter blood and anticoagulate it before it is centrifuged and reinfused if needed.

Indications: Major blood loss in surgery > 20%, rare blood groups, Jehovah's witness', elective caesarean section, post-operative salvage in orthopaedics and predicted blood loss of 500–1000 ml.

Cautions: Contraindicated in bowel or cancer surgery due to contamination, in elective surgery patients need to give informed consent.

Other considerations: 20% reduction in donor blood exposure, transfuse within 4 hours of processing, label bags in theatre.

EPO

Introduction: Recombinant preparations of EPO administered SC or IV. Exists as alfa and beta (epoetin) and darbepoetin alfa.

Indications: Anaemia in renal disease or MDS, 3 weeks prior to PAD or in elective orthopaedic surgery to optimise certain patients.

Cautions: Uncontrolled hypertension following administration, EPO receptor +ve cancer growth, red cell aplasia, risk of VTE increased if Hct > 0.35%.

Other considerations: Dosing, scheduling and indication varies across different preparations.

Iron infusion

Introduction: Oral iron generally preferred but IV iron is quicker acting and used in those failing or intolerant of oral iron.
Indications: As above plus those pre-operatively who do not want a transfusion or in conjunction with EPO.
Cautions: Severe reactions to iron products, give pre-medication beforehand, contraindicated in first trimester of pregnancy.
Other considerations: Newer preparations often given more rapidly than older ones and can repeat the dose if needed.

Desmopressin

Introduction: Causes the release of endogenous factor VIIIc and VWF and can be administered several ways.
Indications: Prevention or treatment in mild haemophilia, type 1 VWD, bleeding with uraemia and platelet dysfunction.
Cautions: Hyponatraemia, repeated doses less effective, monitoring of levels to assess response but requires specialist lab.
Other considerations: Check a DDAVP level and factor VIII to assess the response and guide further treatment.

Recombinant factor VII

Introduction: Activates clotting via extrinsic pathway via TF exposure from endothelial damage, used in major haemorrhage as last option.
Indications: Major haemorrhage which is unresponsive, bleeding in haemophilia A or B with inhibitors, used in severe surgical bleeds off label.
Cautions: Risk of reaction in inhibitor patients, thrombotic risk once haemostasis achieved, won't work if acidotic in major haemorrhage.

TPO-RA

Introduction: Mimics which increase platelet production by megakaryocyte stimulation. Can be given SC or oral.
Indications: Treatment of ITP, newer data in aplastic anaemia and MDS with some centres using them for these indications already.
Cautions: VTE risk to manage once platelets in range, bone marrow fibrosis and reactions.
Other considerations: Flexible dosing schedule based on numerous factors which can help to titrate them.

Tranexamic acid

Introduction: Used widely in prevention and treatment of haemorrhage, works by inhibition of fibrinolysis, cheap and widely available.

Indications: Trauma, major haemorrhage, obstetric surgery, patients with mild bleeding disorders pre-surgery, ICB.

Cautions: Haematuria due to risk of clot retention. Once haemostasis achieved manage thrombotic risk accordingly.

Other considerations: Not plasma derived, reduces risk of transfusion by 30%, available oral, IV, mouthwash and topical.

Transfusion Reactions

Acute

ABO Incompatibility

Introduction: Acute transfusion reactions occur rapidly and within the first 24 hours of transfusion. ABO incompatibility is a transfusion which is ABO major mismatched and is life threatening even with only a few ml of blood.

Epidemiology: 2000 near misses since 2016. 2 deaths due to ABO incompatible red cell transfusions in 2022 according to SHOT report. 30% of ABO incompatibility end in significant morbidity and 10% end in mortality.

Causes: Transfusion of donor red cells which are incompatible with the recipient ABO grouping. Patients may be mismatched and have no reaction i.e., Group O cells given to Group A recipient if the group is not known or in emergencies when Group A is not available. Rarely can happen with high titre anti-A or B plasma or platelets. Often the cause is human error at some stage in the transfusion timeline.

Signs/symptoms: Pain at transfusion site, abdominal pain, tachycardia, hypotension, bleeding from cannula, shortness of breath, sense of impending doom. Other symptoms like chest pain or fever can also occur.

Pathophysiology: The incorrectly transfused red cells react with the patients anti-A or B antibodies in the plasma causing severe intravascular haemolysis of the donor cells, proinflammatory cytokine release, further widespread haemolysis occurs with consumptive coagulopathy and renal failure. This underlying pathological process leads to shock and severe hypotension and ultimately cardiovascular collapse.

Diagnosis: Generally made following patient symptoms and identification of incorrect unit for patient.

Blood results: Haemolytic anaemia with AKI, hepatic dysfunction and raised LDH, DIC picture, haemoglobinuria, DAT +ve.

Initial management:
1. STOP THE TRANSFUSION and have someone check the unit labels and patient ID.
2. ABC assessment and get help as soon as possible if needed.
3. Resus care if needed.
4. IVF and supportive care.
5. Once safe and patient stable CALL TRANSFUSION LAB or ask someone to do so for you as there may be other units being issued incorrectly.
6. Ideally remove cannula and place new one to prevent any further blood being flushed through but maintain access as best as possible.
7. Return bag and giving set to transfusion lab with all labels and documentation.
8. SEEK EXPERT HELP EARLY from on call transfusion lead.
9. Send the relevant investigations below.

Treatment of complications:

Hypotension: IVF, ITU support and if needed inotropic support. Not licensed but consideration of interleukin inhibitory agents such as tocilizumab and high dose steroids for those with cytokine release syndrome type picture.

Renal failure: IVF and early renal support and input, may need dialysis to support through initial large haemolytic episode.

Haemolysis: High dose steroids have been used as well as plasma exchange with FFP.

DIC: Daily clotting and treat bleeding with either plasma, fibrinogen, cryo or platelets based on blood counts.

Investigations: FBC, coagulation screen, DAT, liver function, LDH, renal function, conjugated and unconjugated bilirubin, MSU for haemoglobinuria, repeat grouping and antibodies after stabilised, review a blood film, blood cultures, reticulocyte, haptoglobin.

Supportive care: Thromboprophylaxis, IVF, high flow oxygen, may need CVVH for a long time to prevent kidney damage.

Follow up procedure: Review at local transfusion committee, report to SHOT, lookback investigation and review of each step leading to problem, retraining of transfusion staff and clinicians, ensure use of LIMS system adhered to for safe transfusion issuing.

Anaphylaxis

Introduction: Anaphylaxis to blood products is rare but occurs largely the same way that anaphylaxis to medications does. It is more common in patient with IgA deficiency and in patients receiving plasma or platelets though can occur from any blood product.
Epidemiology: Allergic reactions with hypotension requiring adrenaline reported as 34 by SHOT in 2022. 0 deaths.
Causes: IgA deficiency or conditions associated with IgA deficiency such as Coeliac disease.
Signs/symptoms: Lip swelling or angioedema, rash, fever, tachycardia, stridor, tachypnoea, hypoxia, hypotension.
Pathophysiology: Either IgE mediated through basophils following antigen stimulation and previous exposure or if no previous exposure non-IgE mediated via direct stimulation of mast cells or other immune complexes such as complement. This causes release of inflammatory cytokines and interleukins causing bronchospasm, angioedema and hypotension.
Diagnosis: From clinical signs and symptoms and response to adrenaline. Raised serum tryptase levels can help aid the diagnosis.
Blood results: Raised serum tryptase and acute phase proteins, LDH likely will be raised, signs of haemolysis not common.
Initial management:
1. STOP THE TRANSFUSION and have someone check the unit labels and patient ID.
2. ABC assessment and get help as soon as possible if needed from ITU/anaesthetics for airway support.
3. Resus care for anaphylaxis with 0.5 ml of 1:1,000 IM adrenaline.
4. IVF, supportive care and steroids and antihistamines in addition to adrenaline.
5. Once safe and patient stable CALL TRANSFUSION LAB or ask someone to do so for you.
6. Ideally remove cannula and place new one to prevent any further blood being flushed through but maintain access as best as possible.
7. Return bag and giving set to transfusion lab with all labels and documentation.
Investigations: FBC, DAT, review blood film, serum tryptase, IgA levels once out of acute episode, blood cultures, complement levels, CXR, ABG if hypoxic.
Supportive care: Thromboprophylaxis, antihistamines and steroids for symptoms, review other medication.
Follow up procedure: Review at local transfusion committee, report to SHOT, lookback investigation and review of each step leading to problem, refer to immunologist for investigations for IgA deficiency, ensure all involved in transfusion are BLS trained, may need IgA deficient donors for those with IgA deficiency or SD-FFP, patient education, patient alert card and notify NHSBT.

Transfusion Associated Circulatory Overload

Introduction: Circulatory overload within 6 hours of a transfusion commonly manifesting as pulmonary oedema and respiratory distress, more common in the elderly or small patients from any blood product.

Epidemiology: 1:20,000 risk, but higher in certain groups. SHOT report 160 total and 8 cases of mortality due to TACO in 2022.

Causes: Older patient, often > 70-years-old, history of CCF or respiratory condition, low BMI, history of numerous infusions or transfusion prior to symptoms, multiple transfusions in the same day, renal failure, malnourished, not assessing in between transfusions.

Signs/symptoms: SOB, raised JVP, CXR showing pulmonary oedema, tachypnoea, hypoxia, peripheral oedema, hypertension, tachycardia.

Pathophysiology: Inability to compensate for the additional volume of fluid into the closed cardiovascular system leads to endothelial leak of fluid as well as reduced cardiac output and as a result peripheral oedema and pleural effusions.

Diagnosis: Clinical diagnosis of signs and symptoms, CXR findings and transfusion within 6 hours of symptom onset.

Blood results: Often normal, BNP may be raised and CXR would show signs of pulmonary oedema or pleural effusions.

Initial management:
1. STOP THE TRANSFUSION and have someone check the unit labels and patient ID.
2. ABC assessment and get help as soon as possible.
3. Resus care with high flow oxygen.
4. IV diuretics and catheter for urine output monitoring if needed.
5. Once safe and patient stable CALL TRANSFUSION LAB or ask someone to do so for you.
6. Return bag and giving set to transfusion lab with all labels and documentation.
7. Send relevant investigations.

Investigations: CXR, ECHO, ABG, monitor urine output, renal function, BNP, troponin, strict fluid balance, daily weights.

Supportive care: Continued diuretics, review medications, may need CPAP, renal review for dialysis and UF, ECHO and cardio review.

Follow up procedure: As above.

Transfusion Related Acute Lung Injury

Introduction: TRALI is a relatively uncommon complication, often from plasma-based products or platelets, leading to SOB and hypoxia because of donor antibodies from the blood products interacting with pulmonary granulocytes within 6 hours of transfusion.
Epidemiology: Patients if spotted early and supported by ITU can make full recovery and often do well. 5 cases in 2022 SHOT report.
Causes: Higher incidence from female plasma donors, high titre anti-A and B products, underlying lung pathology or infection.
Signs/symptoms: Symptoms usually occur quicker than TACO, often within 2 hours, SOB, productive frothy sputum, hypoxia, JVP normal, hypotension, fevers, occasionally associated cytopaenias.
Pathophysiology: Granulocytes within the lung react with donor antibodies leading to inflammatory cytokine release and endothelial leak from pulmonary tissue. Cause non-cardiogenic pulmonary oedema, fevers and hypotension.
Diagnosis: Often made on clinical signs and symptoms with associated CXR appearance showing bilateral pulmonary infiltrates. Unlike TACO, fever and rigors may occur though not very common.
Blood results: Neutropaenia and monocyotpaenia, often BNP and ECHO normal compared to TACO. May show rise in acute phase proteins such as CRP, ESR and ferritin.
Initial management:
1. STOP THE TRANSFUSION and have someone check the unit labels and patient ID.
2. ABC assessment and get help as soon as possible ideally with ITU/anaesthetic airway support.
3. Resus care with high flow oxygen and IVF.
4. Once safe and patient stable CALL TRANSFUSION LAB or ask someone to do so for you.
5. Return bag and giving set to transfusion lab with all labels and documentation.
6. Send relevant investigations.
Investigations: CXR, ECHO, ABG, FBC, blood film, BNP, troponin, strict fluid balance, daily weights, blood cultures, CT chest.
Supportive care: Ongoing ITU care with NIV or invasive ventilation, trials of steroids have showed no benefit, respiratory review, may need antibiotics if associated CAP, thromboprophylaxis.
Follow up procedure: Review at local transfusion committee, report to SHOT, lookback investigation and review of each step leading to problem, improved pre-transfusion or inter-transfusion assessments by transfusion staff, inform NHSBT and donor will need to be removed from further donations.

Bacterial Infection

Introduction: Bacterial infection of a blood product, more likely platelets, leading to profound septic shock. Although rare the most likely causative agent is a skin contaminant due to incorrect sterilisation and drying prior to donation procedure.

Epidemiology: Of the 115 reported suspected bacterial infections to SHOT, none were confirmed as bacterial infection in 2022.

Causes: Rare due to screening at donation and post-donation but much more common with platelets due to storage temperature.

Signs/symptoms: Often occurring very quick from starting transfusion, rapid onset of fever, rigors, hypotension, impaired consciousness, and signs of severe sepsis and shock.

Pathophysiology: The same as severe septic shock due to IV infusion of a blood transfusion containing a pathogen leading to endotoxin release causing vasodilation and circulatory collapse. Often it is a skin contaminant rather than from the blood donation itself.

Diagnosis: Based on symptoms above, particularly fever rising above 2°C from baseline, rigors, loss of consciousness. Rise in CRP can aid diagnosis but +ve bacterial culture from patient matching donation via molecular typing confirms diagnosis.

Blood results: Rise in CRP, +ve cultures, DIC picture in some, raised procalcitonin, AKI, raised LDH and lactate.

Initial management:
1. STOP THE TRANSFUSION and have someone check the unit labels and patient ID as well as VISUALLY INSPECTING the bag.
2. ABC assessment and get help as soon as possible ideally with ITU/anaesthetic airway support.
3. Resus care with high flow oxygen, IVF, BLOOD CULTURES and BROAD-SPECTRUM ABX with gram +ve and -ve cover.
4. Once safe and patient stable CALL TRANSFUSION LAB or ask someone to do so for you.
5. Return bag and giving set to transfusion lab with all labels and documentation.
6. Send relevant investigations.

Investigations: Blood cultures peripherally as well as from the cannula and the donation, MSU, CXR, CRP, FBC, renal function.

Supportive care: Sepsis 6 management with ITU support for inotropes and microbiology for treatment of organism, thromboprophylaxis.

Follow up procedure: Review at local transfusion committee, report to SHOT, lookback investigation and review of each step leading to problem, ensure storage conditions for products working, traceability of donor and check them, improve cleaning and drying preparation at donation centres.

Febrile Non-Haemolytic Transfusion Reactions

Introduction: Mild transfusion reaction associated with fever due to donor white cells causing cytokine release.

Epidemiology: More common with red cells but can happen with any product. Generally, most are mild reactions.

Causes: Can happen with any blood product, more common in patients undergoing multiple unit transfusion, less common now due to leucodepletion but still occurs relatively frequently.

Signs/symptoms: Fever, myalgia, rigor, occasionally nausea and mild SOB.

Mild FNHTR: Temperature rises but < 2°C from baseline.

Moderate FNHTR: Temperature rise > 2°C from baseline or > 39°C.

Severe FNHTR: As for moderate but both > 2°C from baseline and > 39°C with symptoms.

Pathophysiology: Commonly due to cytokine build up and storage from blood products with high white cell counts that have not been adequately leucodepleted.

Diagnosis: Made by assessment of clinical symptoms and observations.

Blood results: Often normal.

Initial management:

1. STOP THE TRANSFUSION and have someone check the unit labels and patient ID.
2. ABC assessment and call for help as needed.
3. Supportive care with paracetamol and other pre-medication such as hydrocortisone and chlorphenamine.
4. Once temperature improved restart the transfusion at a slower rate.
5. If further spikes or high spikes then may need to stop the transfusion, clinical review of patient and inform the transfusion lab.

Investigations: Often nothing is needed if mild except observation.

Supportive care: IV paracetamol, hydrocortisone and chlorphenamine. Antiemetic if nausea and pethidine if uncontrolled fever and rigors.

Follow up procedure: Review at local transfusion committee and if severe and persisting report to SHOT.

Delayed

Delayed Haemolytic Transfusion Reaction

Introduction: Delayed transfusion reactions are classified as any reaction occurring 24 hours or more after a transfusion has been administered and can occur up to 2 weeks after transfusion. A delayed haemolytic transfusion reaction occurs due to red cell alloantibody generation leading to a haemolytic anaemia of varying severity.

Epidemiology: More common in pregnancy or multiple pregnancies, multiple transfused patients i.e., patient with sickle cell anaemia, underlying autoimmune condition such as SLE may predispose, ABO incompatible transfusion, previous major haemorrhage treatment. 29 reported in SHOT 2022 report with antibodies detected in 27 cases.

Causes: Most common antibodies are Jk^a and Jk^b from the Kidd group and RhE from the Rh group. In theory most antibodies can cause a reaction though these are the most common in term of clinically significant antibodies.

Signs/symptoms: Symptomatic anaemia, jaundice, dark urine, pale stools, occasionally fever or reduced urine output in severe cases.

Pathophysiology: Antibody develops often over time and is below the limit of detection prior to transfusion. On transfusion the antigen on the red cell which corresponds to the antibody reactivates via alloimmunisation and haemolysis ensues.

Diagnosis:

- Symptoms.
- Transfusion history.
- Haemolytic picture.
- Presence of a new detectable recognised antibody.

Blood results: Haemolytic anaemia picture i.e., raised LDH, retics and bilirubin, anaemia. DAT +ve, haemoglobinuria.

Initial management: IVF and send investigations listed below. Specialist transfusion help, inform transfusion lab. Avoid further transfusions unless necessary in the acute period. If severe a trial of high dose steroids as per AIHA guidelines may be needed or in life threatening scenarios, consider IVIG or plasma exchange.

Investigations: FBC, reticulocytes, DAT, blood film review, LDH, renal function, haptoglobins, repeat group and screen with extended antibody screen sent to NHSBT reference lab, red cell phenotyping.

Supportive care: IVF to prevent AKI, folic acid, thromboprophylaxis, oxygen if hypoxic.

Follow up procedure: Transfusion alternatives in the future, antibody card to empower the patient, report to SHOT and discuss a local transfusion committee, red cell phenotyping going forward for blood -ve for the corresponding antigen.

Post-Transfusion Purpura

Introduction: Autoimmune mediated thrombocytopaenia commonly by the HPA-1a antibody following the transfusion of red blood cells, leading to bleeding around 1-week post-transfusion.

Epidemiology: Rare, more common in HPA-1a -ve women exposed to HPA-1a +ve antigen in first pregnancy.

Signs/symptoms: Petechial rash, mucosal bleeding, GI bleeding, can present with ICB in severe circumstances, symptoms of haemolytic anaemia if red cells affected also.

Pathophysiology: HPA-1a antigen -ve person is sensitised by HPA-1a antigen, commonly when -ve mothers have a fetus who is +ve, leading to antibody generation. Exposure to HPA antigen during pregnancy or transfusion leads to antibody generation. Red blood cells containing small platelet antigens or fragments can then reinitiate the exposure and antigen production leading to destruction of their own antigen -ve platelets consequently. Anti-HPA-1a by far the most common antibody but others such as anti-HPA-5b recognised.

Diagnosis:
- Thrombocytopaenia.
- Transfusion within the last 2 weeks.
- Presence of a new detectable recognised anti-platelet antibody.

Blood results: Isolated thrombocytopaenia which is often moderate to severe. Can have a bystander reaction affecting red cells then a haemolytic anaemia may also be seen.

Initial management: Manage any bleeding with adjuncts such as TXA, specialist transfusion help, inform transfusion lab. IVIG is the treatment of choice with or without high dose steroids.

Investigations: FBC, reticulocytes, DAT, blood film review, repeat group and screen with extended antibody screen sent to NHSBT reference lab for anti-platelet antibodies and if needed genotyping, rule out lymphadenopathy or other underlying causes such as viral infection.

Supportive care: Folic acid, TXA to prevent or treat bleeding, avoid platelet transfusion unless necessary due to life threatening bleeding or surgery needed etc, VTE prophylaxis once suitable.

Follow up procedure: Transfusion alternatives in the future, antibody card to empower the patient, report to SHOT and discuss a local transfusion committee, washed red cells or HPA-1a antigen or whichever antibody is implicated -ve blood, discuss with obstetrics team in the future to manage pregnancies.

Transfusion Associated GvHD

Introduction: Rare but often fatal complication of passenger lymphocytes from predominantly red blood cell transfusion, though can occur in any product, in heavily immunocompromised patients resulting in lymphocyte expansion, engraftment and symptoms of graft versus host disease following the transfusion.

Epidemiology: Incredibly rare and only in risk groups below, prevented by leucodepletion and irradiation. 1 reported since 2000.

Causes/risk factors: Following allograft transplant, following T-cell depleting chemotherapy i.e., fludarabine or bendamustine, certain conditions and associated therapies such as AA with ATG, blood product from closely related HLA haplotype, neonates yet to develop T-cell mediated immunity, IUT, inherited condition affecting T-cells unable to identify foreign antigens. These patients should have irradiated products and TA-GvHD happens in those who should get irradiated products but don't get them.

Signs/symptoms: Symptoms tend to develop 1–2 weeks post transfusion and are like those of GvHD seen in allograft such as rash, fever, diarrhoea and GI symptoms, deranged liver function and any other organ which is typically affected by GvHD can be compromised.

Pathophysiology: Passenger lymphocytes are not recognised as foreign by innate immune system of immunocompromised patient and allowed to proliferate and recognise the recipients HLA-type as foreign and therefore mount an immune/inflammatory response. Proliferation of T-effector cells and infiltration into organs occurs exacerbating the immune response and amplifying damage.

Diagnosis:

- History of transfusion of non-irradiated product in a high-risk individual.
- Biopsy of the affected organ showing lymphocyte infiltration from the donor matched by molecular studies or DNA.

Blood results: Depending on organ affected will lead to the relevant abnormal bloods. Pancytopaenia may occur also if marrow aplasia.

Initial management:

1. If noted early enough STOP THE TRANSFUSION.
2. ABC approach and stabilise patient though likely effects won't occur until days later.
3. Transfer unit and return giving set to lab.
4. Admit patient and discuss with a specialist in transfusion and transplant haematology on next steps. Treatment is often unsuccessful but consists of the same treatment of acute GvHD such as high dose steroids, anti-TNF therapy, immunomodulatory drugs and ECP if needed.

Investigations: Biopsy crucial for diagnosis.

Supportive care: As per GvHD.

Follow up procedure: Training of haematology and transfusion staff to ensure understanding, report to SHOT and internal transfusion committee, ensure LIMS system is working, systematic review of errors leading to issue and administration of blood, communication between blood banks, patient alert cards, centralising these patients records on NHSBT systems.

Blood Borne Viruses and Infections

For the exam mention you would "Use the JPAC geographical risk index and donor selection guidelines for deciding on additional viral testing needed for those who have travelled or may have additional risk factors for acquiring BBV".

HIV

Introduction: HIV 1 and 2 are an RNA virus transmitted through infected blood or bodily fluid.

Epidemiology: Prevalence has reduced thanks to the introduction of patient education, reduced stigma around sexual health testing and the introduction of HAART and PREP. 4 cases since 1980 identified by SHOT with last in the early 2000s. Both due to antigen -ve testing in window period of infection and seroconversion. Estimated risk of HIV entering blood donation pool is 1:10,000,000. Risk of missing detection of 1 infection within the window period occurring once in 14 years of screening.

Prevention: Donor selection questionnaires and deferral of donation, all donors have HIV NAT for HIV 1 and 2 RNA detection.

Window period: NAT 10–30 days and antigen/antibody testing 18–90 days.

Testing: Anti-HIV 1 and 2 NAT for RNA is mandatory.

Who is screened: All new donors and old donors at every subsequent donation.

Symptoms of infection: Signs of seroconversion such as night sweats, painful lymphadenopathy weight loss or infection.

Diagnosis: Genotyping and molecular matching of HIV RNA from donor, blood product and recipient following transfusion.

Follow up procedure: Look-back investigation of donations or transfusions in the last 3 years, counselling and testing for the recipient and any sexual contacts as well as for the donor, trace any other blood donation from the donor for other recipients, virology referral and HIV and sexual health input.

Hepatitis B

Introduction: Hepatitis B is a DNA virus transmitted through infected blood or bodily fluid.

Epidemiology: More common in eastern populations or donors from those endemic areas. 15 cases of transfusion associated hepatis B infection from 1996–2022 all due to donation in the window period between infection and +ve hepatitis B virus serology. Estimated risk of virus entering the blood donation pool is 1:1,500,000. Risk of missing detection of 1 infection within the window period occurring once in 6 months of screening.

Prevention: As above plus serology testing for hepatitis B virus on all new donors and each subsequent donation.

Window period: On average 90 days but can be up to 150.

Testing: HBsAg to indicate if current or previous infection is mandatory. HBV NAT has been introduced and HBV anti-core antibody currently being rolled out to assess for previous cleared HBV infection.

Who is screened: All donors at each donation.

Symptoms of infection: May be asymptomatic if clear virus and no active infection, fevers, jaundice, cirrhosis or signs of decompensated liver failure, bleeding if severe and complications of chronic liver disease such as varices or increased risk of HCC.

Diagnosis: As above for HIV but with HBV genotyping.

Follow up procedure: As above plus consultation with hepatology and initiation of treatment such as tenofovir or entecavir.

Hepatitis C

Introduction: Hepatitis C is an RNA virus transmitted through infected blood or bodily fluid.

Epidemiology: 150–200,000,000 cases worldwide, higher risk in Eastern populations. Only 2 cases reported and confirmed from 1996–2021 as transfusion acquired HCV infection. Risk of HCV infected blood donation entering donor pool is 1:25,000,000. Risk of missing detection of 1 infection within the window period occurring once in 22 years.

Prevention: As above as well as HCV testing.

Window period: Average 2–3 months for +ve serology but ranges from 2 weeks to 6 months.

Testing: Anti-HCV antigen and HCV RNA NAT are mandatory.

Who is screened: All donors at each donation.

Symptoms of infection: More aggressive than HBV with patient more likely to develop cirrhosis or HCC. Treatment is much more pressing than in HBV which many patients will clear on their own.

Diagnosis: As above but with HCV genotyping.

Follow up procedure: As above but treatment initiation more pressing due to risk of cirrhosis and other complications of chronic liver disease. Treatment is with direct-acting antivirals (DAA) such as ribavirin, sofosbuvir or combination therapy.

Hepatitis E

Introduction: RNA virus spread via faecal-oral route i.e., from contaminated food or water.

Epidemiology: More prevalent than first thought with 10–15% of UK having +ve serology for HEV antibodies suggesting previous infection. 15 cases of proven HEV infection from transfused blood product from 1996–2022.

Prevention: As above.

Window period: On average 6 weeks but ranges from 2–9 weeks.

Testing: Testing for HEV is not mandatory as per NHSBT however recommendations form SaBTO in 2016 lead to all donations being tested for serology and those +ve tested for viraemia via NAT.

Who is screened: All donors at each donation.

Symptoms of infection: Acute hepatitis symptoms which tends to self-resolve with lower risk of chronic liver disease, though immunocompromised are at risk of more severe hepatitis and chronic liver disease as a result.

Diagnosis: As above but HEV molecular genotyping.

Follow up procedure: As above plus looking for source of infection and accountability/traceability for public health concerns i.e., infected meat.

HTLV-1 and 2

Introduction: RNA viruses which affect T-cells, which is spread via infected blood or bodily fluid.

Epidemiology: Significantly more common in Japan and Africa than Europe. Risk of infection from blood product is almost zero due to leucodepletion and serological testing in the UK. Only 2 transfusion associated infections before1996.

Prevention: As above, leucodepletion and screen for antibodies against HTLV-1 and 2.

Window period: On average 2 months but can vary.

Testing: Anti-HTLV 1 and 2 antibody screening.

Who is screened: All new donors on first donation as well as if any increased risk at subsequent donations.

Symptoms of infection: Risk of ATLL development in around 3% of infected in HTLV-1, asymptomatic in many, some may have lymphadenopathy, splenomegaly, weight loss, can develop HTLV associated myelopathy leading to profound neurological decline, gait abnormalities and spastic paresis.

Diagnosis: As above but molecular genotyping for HTLV-1 or 2.

Follow up procedure: As above plus monitoring for progression to ATLL can be considered.

vCJD

Introduction: Infective prion acquired from ingestion of infected beef leading to spongiform encephalopathy.

Epidemiology: 177 cases of vCJD in the UK following the epidemic in 1996. Reported 4 cases of transfusion associated vCJD infection identified of which 3 died due to complications related to vCJD infection.

Prevention: No screening tests at present for vCJD. Leucodepletion, exclusion of blood donor who have received a transfusion from 1980 onwards, importation of plasma for patients born after 1996 and importation of SD-FFP for patients with TTP undergoing PLEX.

Window period: Years to decades. Hugely variable.

Symptoms of infection: Asymptomatic for years. Early onset dementia, psychosis, neurological plaque formation with characteristic MRI signs.

Diagnosis: As above but for vCJD. Biopsy proven prion disease and transfusion history with +ve blood product.

Follow up procedure: As above but acting quickly to assess if other products are affected as the consequences of infection likely fatal.

CMV

Introduction: Herpes family virus which is transmitted through infected blood or bodily fluid.

Epidemiology: 40–50% of people in the UK affected and long-term asymptomatic carriers.

Prevention: Leucodepletion generally sufficient. CMV -ve donors for high-risk patients.

Testing: CMV serology and if +ve consider DNA NAT.

Who is screened: Only products required for high-risk donors. Not routinely done on all donations.

Symptoms of infection: Often not a problem in immunocompetent. Immuno-compromised or neonates can lead to severe infections and pneumonitis which can be life threatening so certain groups need CMV -ve blood such as neonates, IUT or pregnant women.

Diagnosis: Hard to distinguish between previous infection and transfusion related.

Follow up procedure: As above and consider treatment in immunosuppressed such as letermovir.

Others

Syphilis: Bacterial infection. Antibody serology testing on all donations. No cases of infection from transfusion since 1996.

Malaria: Only 2 cases since 1996. Defer based on travel history and antibody serology for those high risk.

WNV: Common in Africa and Asia with 2-week window. Defer donors who have travelled to area within 28 days or NAT screening earlier.

T. Cruzi: Common to South America. Defer donors who have travelled to endemic country or NAT testing. No cases of transfusion transmission.

Indications for Irradiated Products

Below is a list of those at increased risk of TA-GvHD and therefore who require irradiated blood products. All products in the UK must receive a minimum of 25Gy to be considered adequately irradiated.

Indication	Timeframe for irradiated products
Hodgkin lymphoma	Receive irradiated products lifelong
Purine analogue chemotherapy or ATG	Receive irradiated products lifelong
Allograft stem-cell transplant	From when conditioning chemotherapy begins until 6 months post-transplant, GvHD prophylaxis has been stopped with no signs of GvHD and total lymphocyte count > 1 × 10⁹/L. Consider lifelong in those with chronic GvHD
Autograft stem-cell transplant	From start of conditioning chemotherapy until 3 months post stem-cell reinfusion. If TBI has been used in conditioning regime, then irradiated products for 6 months post-stem cell reinfusion
AA patients	As above for ATG or if HLA-selected platelets and granulocyte infusions
IUT and neonates	Red cells should be irradiated and used within 24 hours of irradiation for both and platelets for IUT. Red cells should be no older than 5 days. Irradiated products should be used for 6 months after **due date** not actual birth date
Inherited T-cell immunodeficiency disorders	Receive irradiated products lifelong if severe. If cardiac surgery required, then check T-cell subsets and if > 30% naïve T-cells and normal total number then no need to irradiate in neonates. If > 2-years-old requiring cardiac surgery and T-cell immunodeficiency disorder is not severe then no need to irradiate
Stem cell donors either PBSC or BM	7 days before donation and until the day of donation
First or second-degree relative	All should be irradiated before infusion even in healthy individual
Granulocytes	All are irradiated prior to infusion
CAR-T cell therapy	As for autograft unless other indication i.e., previous fludarabine etc.

Guideline:
https://onlinelibrary.wiley.com/doi/full/10.1111/bjh.17015

Major Haemorrhage Protocols

Adult

Definition: This may be hard to judge so many argue that in practice apply the principle of "bleeding with haemodynamic compromise or significant bleeding with no sign of stopping" when activating a major haemorrhage protocol. Definitions include:
- Blood loss of 1 blood volume in 24 hours.
- Bleeding of 150 ml/minute.
- Blood loss of 50% in 3 hours.

Teams involved:
- Ward team or A and E.
- Haematology on call.
- Transfusion lab.
- Surgical teams.
- Porters.
- Interventional radiology.

Initial steps:
1. ABCDE and put out major haemorrhage call.
2. Attempt to ascertain cause if time.
3. Bloods for FBC, electrolyte coagulation, fibrinogen, VBG, LDH and if possible, TEG or ROTEM.
4. TXA if within 3 hours of trauma 1g IV stat followed by 1g TDS.
5. Often O- blood available in A and E fridge which can be used.
6. Request RBC and FFP in a ratio know higher than 2:1 and often 1:1 to avoid dilutional coagulopathy. Typically, 4 units RBC and 4 FFP.
7. Consider drug history, is there a reversal agent for any drugs contributing to bleeding such as PCC to use straight.
8. Reassess ABCDE, if bleeding has stopped and resend bloods after each cycle of transfusion. If blood results not available move to secondary steps. If result available, see targets below.

Targets:
Hb: > 70 g/L and if falling to give further RBC.
Platelets: > 75 × 10^9/L.
FGN: > 1.5 × 10^9/L. Maintain with cryo.
PTR: < 1.5, maintain with FFP 15–20 ml/kg.

Secondary steps:
1. Give further cycle of RBC and FFP as above.
2. Consider 2 pools of cryoprecipitate.
3. Consider a pool of platelets.
4. Consider involvement of surgeons or interventional radiology for assistance now.

Final steps:
1. Continued cycles of RBC and FFP as well as target directed therapy as above.
2. Other sources of FGN considered such as FGN concentrate.
3. Consider recombinant F7a or aprotinin.

Grouping: O- in known O- patient or females under 50 and Kell- if possible, to avoid sensitisation. O+ in men. As soon as ABO grouping known to use ABO matched. Rh and full grouping to follow and can be used once available. ABO grouping to be confirmed on 2 samples.

Complications: Antibody risks long term to the patient, BBV, dilutional coagulopathy, hypothermia and lactic acidosis can impair haemostasis and should be corrected, ionised hypocalcaemia, hyperkalaemia, avoiding TXA in urological bleeding, any transfusion reaction.

Other considerations: Setting you're in and availability of blood, ensuring stock replenished, is it a mass casualty and others arriving who may need products also, escalation to relevant heads of department, other areas which may suffer i.e. theatre or haem day care, holding elective procedures, importance of correct ID and nominating a team leader to run the major haemorrhage, blood warmer if possible to avoid hypothermia, standing down the transfusion lab once done, to consider when to start VTE prophylaxis once haemodynamically stable.

Trials: CRASH-2: Use of TXA in trauma improves outcomes.

Guidelines:
https://onlinelibrary.wiley.com/doi/10.1111/bjh.18275

Obstetrics

Definition: Blood loss of > 1 L in C-section or > 500 ml in vaginal birth. *Moderate:* > 1 L. *Severe:* > 1.5 L.

Major haemorrhage call initiated if > 20% blood volume loss within 3 hours or 150 ml/min.

Differences to above: Ascertaining the cause i.e., placenta praevia or ruptured uterine artery bleed. Surgical management of bleeding may be needed i.e., ligation, cauterisation, compression or emergency C-section and hysterectomy. Uterine contraction with oxytocin or prostaglandins.

Grouping: O- should be given to all unless blood groups known.

Other considerations: As above plus future pregnancy planning and risk from any antibodies formed or pre-existing, paediatricians to be involved if antenatal haemorrhage.

Trials: WOMAN trial: Reduced bleeding deaths and surgical intervention with TXA following PPH.

Paediatrics

Definition: Blood loss of 80 ml/kg in 24 hours, 40 ml/kg in 3 hours or 3 ml/kg/min. Or uncontrollable bleeding with hypovolaemia.

Differences to above: 20 ml/kg of RBC and FFP initially. Repeated as needed. 10 ml/kg of cryo and 1 ml/kg of platelets for persistent bleeding. Consider FGN concentrate or recombinant factor VIIa once 80 ml/kg of RBC have been transfused. TXA to be given at dose of 15 mg/kg. Administer calcium chloride 10% to prevent against ionized hypocalcaemia.

Grouping: O- generally in all. Prioritise females. Irradiated if under 6 months. Group specific once known.

Paeds and obstetrics protocols are adapted from BSH and tertiary centre protocols I have worked at, some variation may exist across hospitals.

Specific Scenarios

Pregnancy

Fetal Maternal Haemorrhage and Anti-D Prophylaxis

I have split this section into 2 as it is quite large. First, I have focused on the risks, screening and management for the RhD -ve mother and in the HDFN section will focus on risk and treatments to the fetus in HDFN.

Introduction: FMH leads to sensitising events which predispose to HDFN, and a significant risk of morbidity and mortality to the fetus. Details on the specific management of HDFN, antibodies which cause it and how to manage the fetus can be found below.

Epidemiology: 1% become sensitised even with anti-D prophylaxis but this has dropped from 15% since anti-D prophylaxis introduced. 1% of women screened have potentially clinically significant red cell alloantibodies.

Risk factors: Can be spontaneous or provoked events. Any antenatal haemorrhage is a risk. Surgical intervention, CVS or amniocentesis, abdominal trauma, ECV, miscarriage, ectopic pregnancy, stillbirth, termination or removal of a molar pregnancy, previous RhD+ transfusion or history of major haemorrhage or multiple transfusions previously.

Screening: ABO and Rh grouping of mother with antibody screening at booking and 28 weeks. If antibody +ve at 28 weeks to screen and quantify every 2 weeks until delivery. Medical history for previous pregnancies or HDFN, previous FMH or sensitising events. All RhD women should be offered routine anti-D prophylaxis. Those with history of HDFN should be seen by fetal medicine specialist before 20 weeks of any future pregnancies.

Bloods: ABO and Rh grouping on all, FBC and coag on those with FMH, Kleihauer test to quantify FMH as well as flow cytometry, red cell antibody screening initially and if +ve then antibody identification at reference NHSBT laboratory, antibody quantification/titre if clinically significant and consider paternal testing also for risk in future pregnancies. CfDNA can be done for Rh c, C, E or Kell antibodies. CfDNA for fetal genotyping for mothers with:

1. A clinically significant antibody.
2. History of HDFN.
3. Father expresses corresponding antigen or status not known.

Complications of FMH: Risk to mother of anaemia, PPH or in severe circumstances major haemorrhage and complicated transfusion in the future. Risk to fetus of HDFN. Risk to future pregnancies due to antibody generation.

Symptoms: Bleeding, abdominal pain, reduced fetal movements, history of trauma.

Diagnosis: Quantify bleed by acid elution, Kleihauer or flow cytometry. More can be found in lab principles section on the specifics behind these tests.

Prophylaxis: All RhD- women with no history of sensitisation offered anti-D at 28 weeks as 1 dose (1500 IU) or 2 dose (500 IU at 28 weeks and 34 weeks. 1 dose regime is more cost effective and convenient for patient).

Treatment: In the event of sensitising event anti-D prophylaxis should be given within 72 hours but can be given up to 10 days.

Bleed of up to 4 ml: 500 IU of anti-D.

> 4 ml: Extra 125 IU of anti-D per 1 ml of fetal cells and follow up testing in 48–72 hours.

> 100 ml: Large IV anti-D dose or infusion and follow up testing as above as well as fetal monitoring.

< 20 weeks sensitising event: 250 IU anti-D minimum, no FMH testing required.

> 20 weeks: 500 IU anti-D minimum + FMH testing required.

Delivery: 500 IU anti-D prophylaxis within 72 hours of delivery in RhD- women with RhD+ fetus confirmed on cord blood.

Intraoperative cell salvage: C-section on RhD- women with RhD+ fetus confirmed on cord blood should receive 1500 IU anti-D.

Follow up: Antibody testing as mentioned below based on risk of HDFN from titre and history of any anti-D prophylaxis as low anti-D titre could be due to passive D. If FMH quantified as > 4 ml and anti-D dose not sufficient to cover than additional dosing is needed and repeat testing at 72 hours since anti-D given (48 hours if given IV).

Guidelines:

https://transfusionontario.org/wp-content/uploads/2020/06/BCSH-Guideline-for-the-use-of-anti-D-immunoglobulin-for-the-prevention-of-HDFN_Trans-Med_2014.pdf

https://onlinelibrary.wiley.com/doi/epdf/10.1111/tme.12299

Haemolytic Disease of the Fetus and Newborn

Introduction: HDFN is a complication of FMH or a sensitising event in a woman leading to alloantibody production against the corresponding blood group antigen of the fetus leading to haemolysis, IUGR and in severe circumstances death. Commonly occurs in RhD- women with RhD+ fetus, though it can occur due to other Rh group and Kell antibodies.

Epidemiology: Since introduction of anti-D prophylaxis mortality has fallen significantly from affecting around 1:2000 births to affecting < 1:50,000 births.

Risk factors: As above for FMH, previous history of HDFN or known red cell antibodies which can cause HDFN.

Screening: As above. Monitoring of baby includes cfDNA which can be done on Rh c/C, E and Kell antigens, USS doppler monitoring of fetal middle cerebral artery (MCA) peak systolic flow done in antibody +ve pregnancies generally every 1–2 weeks and growth monitoring.

Bloods: As above for FMH. Antibody screening and titres. Post-delivery send cord blood for FBC, DAT, LDH, haptoglobin, group and save and crossmatch, antibody screen and titre. CfDNA if possible.

Complications of HDFN: Hyperbilirubinemia and kernicterus, IUGR, renal failure, reduced erythropoiesis, hydrops fetalis, pre-term birth and stillbirth.

Diagnosis:
- Clinical suspicion based on history.
- Cord blood findings.
- Detectable antibodies which are clinically significant for HDFN.
- Dopplers showing raised MCA peak systolic flow.

Antibodies associated: Anti-D, anti-c and anti-K are the most clinically significant. Other associated with HDFN include anti-Jk^a, Fy^a, C and E.

Prevention: Screening, anti-D prophylaxis, high-risk mothers managed in fetal medicine unit, alternatives to transfusion in women of childbearing age.

Treatment: Preventative measures as mentioned, IUT of red cells if dopplers indicate a peak systolic flow > 1.5 mm/Hg.

IUT requirements: Group O- or ABO matched and low titre, -ve for corresponding antigen to the maternal antibody, irradiated, CMV-, plasma removed to increase the haematocrit (often > 0.75), < 5 days old, RhD and Kell -ve, in SAG-M, sickle screen -ve.

Dose: 80 ml/kg is classified as a large volume red cell IUT. 20 ml/kg a smaller top up IUT.

Neonatal exchange requirements: Blood should be ABO matched and low titre, RhD -ve Kell -ve, corresponding antigen -ve, < 5 days old, CMV -ve, irradiated, stored in CPD rather than SAG-M and haematocrit between 0.5–0.6.

Dose: 200 ml/kg of red cells removes 2 neonatal blood volumes and reduced bilirubin by 50% and neonatal red cells by 90%.

Antibody monitoring: All mothers screen at booking and 28 weeks. If antibody detected either do paternal testing of cfDNA of fetus. If confirmed, then test antibody titre and refer to fetal medicine. If high-risk based on antibody titre, then recheck every 2 weeks after 28 weeks until delivery. If a known antibody of significance, then screen for it and titre every month until 28 weeks unless rising which may increase the need for closer screening intervals.

<u>Anti-D</u>: < *4 IU/ml*: Low risk for HDFN, monitor. *4–15 IU/ml*: Moderate risk of HDFN, refer to fetal medicine. > *15 IU/ml*: High risk, refer to fetal medicine.

<u>Anti-c</u>: < *7.5 IU/ml*: Low risk for HDFN, monitor. *7.5–20 IU/ml*: Moderate risk of HDFN, refer to fetal medicine. > *20 IU/ml*: High risk, refer to fetal medicine.

<u>Anti-K</u>: Titre antibody. Titres as low as 1:8 shown to cause fetal anaemia so reasonable to discuss with fetal medicine specialist at this threshold or if rising. If detected, then screen for antibodies to all other Kell blood group antigens. If other antibodies detected discuss with haematology and if symptoms of fetal anaemia picked up or titre > 1:32 to then send to fetal medicine specialist.

Other considerations: Fetal monitoring, paediatricians involved early, time to get blood for IUT often from frozen blood bank in Liverpool so some logistical planning is needed, blood warmer for IUT and exchange, often aim to deliver baby electively at 37 weeks.

Guidelines:
As above and https://www.rcog.org.uk/media/oykp1rtg/rbc_gtg65.pdf

Neonatal Alloimmune Thrombocytopaenia

Introduction: NAIT occurs because of maternal antibodies generated against fetal HPA platelet antigens causing severe thrombocytopaenia leading to increased risk of preterm delivery, ICB, miscarriage and still birth.

Epidemiology: 90% of cases due to HPA-1a antibody.

Risk factors: Previous history of NAIT, known associated antibody, multiply transfused mothers, HPA antigen -ve mother with +ve associated HPA antigen fetus, history of PTP.

Screening: Mothers screened at booking appointment. If known history can titre the relevant known antibody.

Symptoms: Evidence of ICB or neonatal bleeding on doppler USS, purpuric rash postnatal, extensive bleeding from cord.

Bloods: FBC, virology, LFTs, rule out other reactive causes or vaccine history, rule out other thrombocytopaenia syndromes i.e., HELLP.

Complications: ICB is the major cause of morbidity and mortality, but other significant bleeding can occur i.e., intraabdominal.

Diagnosis:
- Neonatal thrombocytopaenia.
- Detectable associated HPA antibody in maternal serum.

Antibodies associated: HPA-1a by far the most common. 3a or 5b the next most common in NAIT.

Treatment:

Maintenance: $> 25 \times 10^9$/L to reduce risk of ICB or life-threatening bleeding though in reality most centres happier with platelet count $> 50 \times 10^9$/L, especially at delivery.

Severe bleeding: $> 100 \times 10^9$/L.

IUT dosing: 10–20 ml/kg for children < 15kg.

Because of risk of further bleeding with IUT IVIG is also recommended antenatally if deemed too risky to proceed with IUT and no contraindication. Post-delivery platelets spontaneously improve in many around 1 month. In those with severe thrombocytopaenia IVIG may be needed with 75% responding to treatment. Role for platelets only in ICB or life-threatening bleeding.

Blood grouping: Platelets should be HPA antigen -ve for the maternal HPA antibody, single donor apheresis, CMV -ve, irradiated and concentrated to contain a platelet count of 2000×10^9/L.

Other considerations: Future pregnancy monitoring, logistical planning of IUT and delivery of hyperconcentrated platelets, elective admission for delivery considered at 37 weeks based on most up to date platelet count.

Guidelines:

https://b-s-h.org.uk/media/2884/2016-neonates-final-v2.pdf

Sickle Cell Anaemia and Haemoglobinopathies

Introduction: Transfusion requirements for haemoglobinopathy patients can be complex either due to antibody generation from multiple transfusions, iron chelation or the specific requirements needed for exchange transfusion.

Epidemiology: 30% of thalassaemia patients develop antibodies. 60% of sickle cell anaemia patients develop antibodies after 200 transfusions.

Complications: Hyperhaemolysis due to red cells antibodies following transfusion leading to donor and recipient red cell destruction. Often 2–3 days after last transfusion and is life threatening. Red cell transfusion contraindicated and often makes it worse. Treatment is with IVIG and high dose steroids.

Blood requirements: Genotyping can be done in those already transfused but extended phenotyping should be done on all before transfusion ideally.

Thalassaemia: ABO matched red cells with extended phenotyping for all Rh antigens and Kell, -ve for any associated alloantibodies and ideally less than 10 days old.

Sickle cell: As above plus HbS -ve (say it in the exam though in reality most donated blood is, unless the donor har trait) and less than 7 days old for exchange.

Antibodies associated: Most commonly Rh and Kell antibodies in both sickle cell anaemia and thalassaemia. Sickle cell anaemia patients are increased risk of rare phenotypes i.e., Ro, which is very hard to completely crossmatch for.

Other considerations: Iron chelation therapy in those who have had multiple transfusions, blood warmers in exchange transfusion, risk of hyperkalaemia and hypocalcaemia in exchange transfusion, logistical planning of units for rare phenotypes from frozen blood bank in Liverpool, transfusion alternatives and restrictive transfusion practice, empower the patient with antibody cards, virology testing pre-transfusion.

Guidelines:
https://onlinelibrary.wiley.com/doi/full/10.1111/bjh.14346

Transplant

Introduction: ABO incompatible stem cell transplants can be recipient mediated, donor mediated or bidirectional with varying severity based on minor or major incomparability. Rh mismatching is a more delayed process and will not be discussed here.

Epidemiology: 25% of matched sibling allografts are ABO mismatched in some way. Haemolysis can occur immediately or over the next 7–14 days following engraftment.

Prevention: Higher risk for BM harvest transplant compared to PBSC. BM harvest collections can be red cell or plasma depleted to remove passenger red cells or antibodies in major or minor mismatches respectively. This is not needed in PBSC provided the product has < 10 ml of red cells. Other preventative measures include having several donors available, though not always possible, informing stem cell lab of ABO mismatch to prepare for changing of groups as well as having relevant blood bank stock.

Symptoms: That of ABO incompatible red cell transfusion if high enough infusion of red cells from stem cell products. Often not the case due to red cell depletion pre-infusion. Commonly patients have haemolytic anaemia picture and high antibody titre once group has switched.

Mismatches:

Major: Recipient plasma contains antibodies against donor red cells which are incompatible.

Donor: A or B. *Recipient*: O. **OR** *Donor*: AB. *Recipient*: O, A or B.

Minor: Donor plasma contains antibodies against recipient red cells which are incompatible.

Donor: O. *Recipient*: A, B or AB. **OR** *Donor*: A or B. *Recipient*: AB.

Minor: Antibodies in the donor and recipient plasma are incompatible with the donor or recipient red cells.

Donor: A. *Recipient*: B. **OR** *Donor*: B. *Recipient*: A.

Transfusion:

Major: Match red cells to recipient (or group O cells if matched not available) and plasma match to donor. Platelets to donor or in AB donor match to recipient.

Minor: The reverse of major.

Bidirectional: Group O red cells for all. Match platelets to recipient. AB plasma for both. If in doubt O red cells can be given for all scenarios above in emergencies. Once crossed over to donor group by IAT grouping then transfuse the group matched blood products as required.

Treatment: Treat as per any intravascular haemolysis.

Most patients just need supportive care i.e., IVF and folic acid though can consider steroids or IVIG in severe life-threatening circumstances.

Monitoring: Monitoring of blood groups by forward and backwards grouping as well as antibody titre if suspected haemolysis can be useful to guide things and rule out other cause of anaemia/haemolysis in the complex setting of allograft transplants.

Complications: As per haemolytic anaemia and ABO incompatible transfusion as well as delayed or reduced engraftment in severe circumstances but this is rare.

Blood Groups

There are over 40 blood groups. Here I have covered the mandatory group testing, most common in terms of antibody generation and any of clinical significance but there are many more.

Group	Antigens within group	Genes	Haplotypes	Clinically significant antibodies?	Problems associated with antibody formation
ABO	A, B or O	ABO	AA, BB, AO, BO, AB, OO	Yes	Acute haemolytic transfusion reactions Post-transplant haemolysis depending on mismatch
Rh	D, c, C, e, E Nearly 50 in total thought the above are the most clinically significant. Others exists which are clinically significant if antibodies develop i.e., Cw	RHD and RHCE	R_1 = CDe R_2 = cDE R_0 = cDe r = cde r' = Cde Weak D: Reduced quantitative expression D Variant: As above and varied D binding sites	Yes	HDFN Delayed transfusion reactions often severe
Kell	K, k, Kp^a, Kp^b, Js^a, Jsb More but these are the most common	KEL	K -ve or +ve K -ve or +ve Kp (a and b) –ve or +ve combinations Js (a and b) –ve or +ve combinations	Yes	HDFN Delayed transfusion reaction in varying severity
Duffy	Fy^a and Fy^b Fy$^{3-6}$ also but only Fy^3 clinically significant	DARC	Fy (a and b) -ve or +ve combinations Fy (a-b-) protective against *P. falciparum* malaria	Yes	Mild HDFN Delayed transfusion reaction in varying severity

Kidd	Jk^a and Jk^b Jk^3 also, but expression largely the same across most populations	SLC14A1	Jk (a and b) -ve or +ve combinations	Yes	Mild HDFN Delayed transfusion reaction in varying severity But often hard to detect. Anti-Jk^3 can cause acute transfusion reactions
Lutheran	Lu^a and Lu^b. More exists but these are the most common for antibody formation	LU	Lu (a and b) -ve and +ve combinations	No	Rarely HDFN and then very mild
MNS	M, N, S and s. Over 30 more of less clinical significance	GYPA, GYPB, GYPE	-ve and +ve combinations of M, N, S and s	Yes	Antibodies are rare but cause severe HDFN and acute and delayed transfusion reactions
P1Pk	P1, P^k or NOR	A4GALT	-ve or +ve combinations of P1, P^k or NOR	No	Very rare and cases of HDFN mild Some variation of expression in certain cancers
Lewis	Le^a and Le^b	FUT3	Le (a and b) -ve and +ve combinations	No	Rare and very mild case of delayed transfusion reaction
Diego	Di^a, Di^b and Wr^a. More which are less clinically significant	SLC14A1	Di (a and b) -ve or +ve combinations and Wr^a -ve or +ve presence	Yes	Generally severe HDFN Severe delayed transfusion reactions Severe acute transfusion reactions for anti-Wr^a

Lab Principles of Transfusion

I would highly advise you take the time to visit your transfusion lab and do these procedures as it is much easier to convey them by doing them first-hand than through text. The transfusion course also goes into a lot of detail, this is just an overview of the basics.

Blood Grouping

Introduction: The basis of transfusion to help determine a patient's ABO and RhD blood group by forward and reverse grouping. Forward grouping assesses the patient red cell antigens and reverse grouping looks at the patient serum antibodies.

When is the test used: For ABO and Rh matching prior to issue of blood products.

How to perform:

1. Collect patient sample in EDTA anticoagulant tube and centrifuge the specimen.
2. Centrifuge the specimen to collect the patient serum and red cells separately and make a 5% suspension of red cells.
3. Add patient red cells to 2 tubes labelled 1 and 2 with anti-A and B reagents which identify A and B blood group (**forward grouping**).
4. Add patient serum 2 tube labelled 3 and 4 with reagent A and B-cells (**reverse grouping**).
5. Centrifuge the sample and resuspended the red cells to observe for agglutination either by eye or via microscopy depending on lab procedure.
6. For RhD grouping make a 5% suspension of patient red cells and add 1 drop of patient red cell to Anti-RhD reagent and then centrifuge.
7. Resuspend and observe. If agglutination, then RhD +ve. Use albumin as a -ve control to test reagents.

Interpretation: Agglutination in the forward group which is the inverse of the reverse group i.e., if the patient red cells in tube 1 agglutinate on addition of anti-A serum and the patient serum added to tube 4 reacts with the reagent B red cells then this is group A. Group O will have no agglutination when the patient red cells are mixed with A and B reagents but will have a reaction in both tubes when the patient serum is mixed with reagent A and B-cells. The reverse will be seen in patients with blood group AB.

Limitations: False agglutination can be observed in old samples, reagents need regular internal and external validation, cross contamination from other antibodies, false +ve in patients with large paraproteinaemia.

Antibody Screening

Introduction: Red cell antibody screening is done prior to transfusion, pregnancy or in those with known antibodies. The goal is to detect the presence of any antibodies in the patient's serum against red cell antigens but does not identify the antibody. Also done on all blood donors to check for the presence of non-ABO antibodies.

When is the test used: Prior to transfusion, during pregnancy or following large FMH i.e., post-natal. It is used to identify antibodies other than those naturally occurring in the patient plasma i.e., non-ABO group antibodies.

How to perform:

1. Collect patient sample in EDTA anticoagulant tube and centrifuge the specimen to collect the plasma.
2. Commercially available group O red cells expressing a variety of other blood group antigens against common acquired red cell antibodies are added to separate tubes. Often 3 or 4 are used.
3. Add the patient serum to the different tubes in equal volumes, often only 1–2 drops.
4. Centrifuge the samples for 15 seconds.
5. Analyse the sample by eye or microscopy for signs of agglutination.

Interpretation: Agglutination is a +ve result for an antibody detected against antigens present on the red cells. You can miss cold reactive antibodies or have a false +ve from non-specific binding. Next step is to then identify the antibody by the IAT and if necessary, quantify it by an antibody titre test.

Limitations: Not always diagnostic and requires antibody identification testing, may miss rare antibodies so in patients with these important to make them well-known to blood transfusion service.

Antibody Identification (IAT)

Introduction: Antibody identification is performed following a +ve antibody screen and is done via the indirect antiglobulin test or IAT. The test uses the patient's plasma against commercially bought red cells with varying known antigen expression profiles to ascertain which antibody is present in the serum. It uses anti-human globulin which binds to patient IgG antibodies at 37°C.

When is the test used: Following identification of a +ve antibody screening test.

How to perform:

1. As for steps 1–5 in antibody screening.
2. Take 1–2 drops of the patient's serum and mix with commercial group O red cell panels with varying other blood group antigen expression.
3. Mix the samples and incubate at 37°C for up to 1 hour and then observe by eye or microscopically for agglutination for cold antibody detection.
4. Wash the cells 3–4 times with PBS to remove any unbound antibody to prevent false -ve.
5. Add 2 drops of AHG and centrifuge. Observe for agglutination by eye or microscopically.
6. Add IgG sensitised cells as +ve control to ensure reagents working.

Interpretation: Based on the agglutination in the various cell panels expressing different antigens you can deduce if a single antibody is present and likely to be causing the pattern of agglutination seen. If not and it could be 2 or more antibodies need to consider enzyme-based assay, absorption/adsorption study or antibody elution.

Limitations: Normally done at NHSBT reference lab so results not immediate, may miss cold antibodies, reaction time is slow with many steps but use of LISS buffer or other reagents can be used to speed this up, cross reactivity of non-specific antibodies either allo or auto which can cause a false +ve test.

DAT

Introduction: A direct antiglobulin test is used when suspecting immune mediated haemolysis which is either cold, warm or mixed in respect of the associated antibody causing haemolysis. The test uses AHG which can be both polyspecific for IgG or C3d for screening and monospecific for any of the above antibodies for confirmation. AHG binds patient red cells with antibodies which are bound to red cell antigens.

When is the test used: After a transfusion reaction, when suspecting AIHA, cord and maternal blood in HDFN and in other haemolytic anaemias which are non-immune as part of the diagnostic work up.

How to perform: (Test tube collection method)

1. Collect blood in EDTA.
2. Wash patient red cells to remove unbound immunoglobulin and complement.
3. Add 1–2 drops of AHG to 1–2 drops of patient red cells and centrifuge sample for 30 seconds.
4. Resuspend the red cell pellet and observe for degree of agglutination from 0–4 on scale.
5. Use a -ve control with patient red cells and albumin instead of AHG.
6. Following a -ve DAT add commercially bought immunoglobulin coated red cells as a +ve control following a -ve DAT.

Interpretation: Assessing for agglutination and the degree of agglutination by eye and microscopy if needed.

IgG +ve: Warm.

C3d +ve: Cold.

IgG and C3d +ve: Mixed or warm so a DaggT should be performed.

A +ve DaggT at room temperature suggest a mixed or cold AIHA unless the antibody titre is < 1:64 in which case it indicates a warm AIHA. Consider an elution or adsorption study and monospecific DAT based on polyspecific results.

Limitations: +ve following transfusion, as many as 1:1000 in the general population have weakly +ve DAT without clinical cause or significance, false +ve in several conditions such as cancer or infection and relies on lab staff interpretation and performing of test so room for human error.

Donath Landsteiner

Introduction: Used following a +ve DAT or in clinical scenarios when indicated to screen for PCH. In patients with symptoms of AIHA, a +ve DAT and Donath Landsteiner test PCH can be diagnosed. Often associated with acute viral infections or atypical bacterial infections. Positivity is due to an IgG cold associated antibody binding to red cells and complement mediated haemolysis on warming.

When is the test used: DAT +ve with mixed or cold picture and a -ve DaggT or low antibody titre (< 1:64), children with haemoglobinuria or haemolysis which is mediated by the cold irrespective of DAT.

How to perform:

1. Collect blood and centrifuge to obtain serum.
2. Label 3 sets of tubes 1–3 and within each set label tubes A, B and C so you have 9 tubes in total. Add patient serum only, patient serum and normal serum and normal serum only to each tube in each set.
3. Add P-positive commercially bought red cells (as the cold antibody often has an affinity to P-antigen) or patient red cells to the serum and then begin incubations below.
4. Incubate 1 tube from each set (i.e., 1A, 2A and 3A) in a water bath at 37°C for 1 hour, another set in an ice bath for 1 hour and the last set in an ice bath for 30 minutes before transfer to water at 37°C for the next 30 minutes.
5. Observe for haemolysis by eye or via microscopy.

Interpretation: Haemolysis observed in tubes with patient serum (with or without normal serum) that have been incubated in an ice bath and then transferred to a 37°C water bath is a +ve result.

Limitations: Labour intensive and specialised lab staff required to run test with multiple steps.

Kleihauer

Introduction: Kleihauer testing, or the acid elution test is used to screen for and estimate FMH via elution of HbF and HbA from fetal and maternal red cells respectively. It is commonly used in screening when FMH is suspected and if +ve further quantification methods such as flow cytometry are utilised to more accurately quantify the FMH. Works on the principle of HbF being more robust to acid elution than HbA and the HbF can then be stained and analysed to see the degree of FMH.

When is the test used: Screening for FMH when indicated, quantification of known FMH, following anti-D treatment to assess.

How to perform:
1. Collect maternal blood in EDTA and mix before diluting in PBS at a dilution of 1:3.
2. Prepare thin blood films from whole blood mixed sample which are dry and fixed with ethanol.
3. Prepare +ve control of fresh cord blood mixed with adult blood and -ve control of blood with low chance of HbF. These controls can often be commercially bought in kits for the test though in house self-prepared controls still exist.
4. Stain the films with an acid dye, commonly Ehrlich's acid haematoxylin, to cause the denaturing of HbA before being washed several times.
5. Films are then stained with a dye such as erythrosine to stain HbF.
6. Films are examined under the microscope using a screening method or quantification method using adjuncts such as a Miler square.

Interpretation: In screening more than 100 adult cells should be seen per high powered field and then 25 lower powered fields examined for presence of HbF. If there are more than 10 HbF cells per low power field proceed to quantification looking at 10,000 cells and use the Mollison equation to estimate FMH. Or use another method such as flow cytometry. Refer for flow is the FMH is greater than 2 ml.

Limitations: In house kits may differ from other labs, time consuming, requires experienced lab staff, low throughput, human error can occur especially in counting and film making, false +ve in patients with HPFH or other haemoglobinopathies.

Flow Cytometry in FMH

Introduction: Flow cytometry uses a more precise and objective method to quantify FMH by IgG monoclonal antibody fluorochrome conjugate binding to RhD +ve red cells from a blood sample.

When is the test used: To quantify a FMH or if a +ve screening in a Kleihauer is estimated > 2 ml. Also, in patients where Kleihauer not appropriate such as HPFH or other haemoglobinopathies where HbF may be raised.

How to perform:
1. EDTA whole blood sample is collected and mixed thoroughly.
2. Wash the sample thoroughly in PBS to remove leucocytes which may give false +ve and centrifuged to remove platelets.
3. Cells are stained using an antibody with high affinity for RhD antigen based on the advised dilution from the reagent and leave to incubate at room temperature in the dark or as per the manufacturer's guidance.
4. Stain +ve controls, often provided commercially, to quantify any background staining from the antibody which is to be subtracted from the patient sample. -ve controls are often known Rh D -ve cells.
5. Run sample controls through flow cytometer and set gating appropriately.
6. Run ideally 2 maternal samples and no fewer than 500,000 events should be observed.

Interpretation: Calculate using the Mollison equation as above based on the % of fetal cells calculated by flow cytometry.

Limitations: More expensive than Kleihauer and requires expert lab technician to run test and clinical scientist or clinician with experience to interpret the test, not all centres have access on site and needs external referral.

Abbreviations and Organisations in Transfusions

A brief overview of the organisations involved in safe transfusion practice.

NHSBT: NHS blood and transplant. Integral part of the blood service for blood donors, recipients, sample testing and processing, sample storage and delivery. Also work with transplant services, diagnostic services in transfusion and develop clinical research.

JPAC: Joint United Kingdom (UK) Blood Transfusion and Tissue Transplantation Services Professional Advisory Committee. Provides guidance on blood and stem cell donation as well as acting as an independent advisory board for UK blood transfusion services.

SHOT: Serious Hazards of Transfusion. Independent reviewer of adverse transfusion events within the UK since 1996. Aims to report on risk and problems associated with transfusion in regular reports to improve transfusion practices and patient safety.

SaBTO: The advisory committee on the Safety of Blood, Tissue and Organs. Committee of healthcare professionals which provide safety measures and advice to trusts and government organisations on best practices for transplant and transfusion.

MHRA: Medicines and Healthcare products Regulatory Agency. Involved in the regulation and reporting of serious adverse reaction or events from blood products or components.

SABRE: Serious Adverse Blood Reactions and Events. MHRA system for reporting adverse transfusion events.

UK NEQAS: United Kingdom National External Quality Assessment Service. Monitors transfusion and blood bank laboratory services by external quality assessment of assays and lab practices. Ensures a set of standards are met which are comparable, safe and reproducible to ensure the best clinical outcomes for patients.

UKAS: United Kingdom Accreditation Service. National accreditation service which is government led to independently assess any organisation, not just healthcare, that provide testing or calibration services.

EBMT: European Society for Blood and Marrow Transplantation. Board of experienced healthcare professionals providing expertise and guidance on transfusion, transplant and cellular therapies.

JACIE: The Joint Accreditation committee ISCT-Europe and EBMT. European accreditation service for hospitals to administer stem cell transplant and cellular therapies.

Haemostasis and Thrombosis

Haemostasis and Thrombosis 214

For this section the structure will differ slightly. For the relevant tests that are described the goal is to describe the assay, how it is used, what may affect it and some of the background behind the assay itself. Conditions mentioned will attempt to follow the same structure as the haematological oncology section. The layout will be in essay format where possible. As some of the special tests have multiple steps, I will list them in a bullet point concise order and then list pitfalls or points of relevance at the end. I have covered the main tests from the BSH guidelines; I have not covered some extra ones which exist in other resources, as these are quite complex and other external resources should be used for them for a clearer understanding.

Basic Coagulation Tests

Activated Partial Thromboplastin Time

Introduction: The APTT is a coagulation test used to screen for problems in the common and intrinsic pathways. It may also be sensitive to inhibitors such as the lupus anticoagulant, but this varies according to reagent sensitivity, so it is worth being familiar with the practice in the lab where you work.

What it measures: Deficiencies in factors V, VIII, IX, XI and XII and prothrombin.

Normal range: Lab values vary but largely 25–35 seconds.

How to perform:
1. Blood collected in blue top sodium citrate to line of tube for appropriate dilution for calcium chelation. In patients with high haematocrit then blood to citrate volumes may need to be adjusted to maintain the same ratio of 9:1.
2. Sample centrifuged to collect plasma from red cells, platelets, and mononuclear cells.
3. APPT reagent containing contact activator (e.g., silica or ellagic acid) and phospholipids added and mixed.
4. Incubate at 37°C.
5. Calcium added, timer started. Sample is measured for the time taken for the initial clot to form. (i.e., first fibrin strands to polymerise).
6. Clot detection is performed by electro-mechanical or photo-optical methods.

Benefits: Quick and easy to perform. No special steps needed. Recognised by multiple specialities and hospitals. Good screening tool for factor deficiencies. Degree of prolongation tends to relate to severity of factor deficiency.

Limitations: Traumatic venepuncture can lead to sample clotting. Does not provide diagnosis. Based on historic understanding of coagulation (classical "waterfall" cascade model) rather than physiological initiation, amplification, and propagation phases of coagulation (cellular based model).

Isolated prolongation: Heparin (perform a thrombin time and anti Xa), incorrect citrate dilution (see above), factor VIII, IX, XI and XII deficiencies (usually needs to be 20–40% deficient to affect APTT), lupus anticoagulant- perform a DRVVT, warfarin or DOACS and specific factor inhibitors.

Reduced by: Incorrect citrate dilution, lab error, sepsis or reactive cause of elevated factor VIII, rarely thrombophilia.

Phrases for the essay: Analysers and reagents should pass internal and external quality assessments and be checked regularly. Analysers and reagents should follow the manufacturer's guidelines for use.

Further reading:
https://practical-haemostasis.com/Screening%20Tests/aptt.html
https://onlinelibrary.wiley.com/doi/full/10.1111/bjh.16776

Prothrombin Time

Introduction: The PT is a coagulation test used to screen for problems with the common and extrinsic pathways.

What it measures: Factors V, VII and X. Fibrinogen and prothrombin also.

Normal range: Lab values vary but largely 9–15 seconds.

How to perform:

1. Blood collected in blue top sodium citrate to line of tube for appropriate dilution for calcium chelation.
2. Sample centrifuged to separate plasma from red cells, platelets and mononuclear cells.
3. PT reagent containing tissue factor, phospholipids and calcium chloride and start timer.
4. Incubate at 37°C.
5. Clot detection is performed by electro-mechanical or photo-optical methods.

Benefits: Quick and easy to perform. No special steps needed. Recognised by multiple specialities and hospitals.

Limitations: Traumatic venepuncture can lead to sample clotting, does not give diagnosis.

Isolated prolongation: Factor VII deficiency, early in warfarin treatment (factor VII has short half-life) and use of DOACS.

Reduced by: Incorrect citrate dilution, lab error, treatment with factor VII.

Further reading:

https://practical-haemostasis.com/Screening%20Tests/pt.html

Combined APTT and PT prolongation: Common pathway factor deficiency, vitamin K deficiency, liver disease, DOACS or high concentration of unfractionated heparin, dilutional coagulopathy, multiple factor deficiencies.

INR: Used to standardise PT across labs to allow for warfarin monitoring based on the result.

Calculated by the patients PT result divided by the geometric mean PT (from 20 healthy donors) squared by the ISI.

The ISI is specific to each thromboplastin reagent used in measuring PT and assess how sensitive it is to deficiencies in vitamin K.

Thrombin Time

Introduction: The TT is a coagulation test used to assess fibrinogen deficiency and dysfunction or thrombin inhibitors.

What it measures: Thrombin and fibrinogen.

Normal range: Lab values vary but 13–15 seconds.

How to perform:

1. Blood collected in blue top sodium citrate to line of tube for appropriate dilution for calcium chelation.
2. Sample centrifuged to collect plasma from red cells, platelets and mononuclear cells.
3. Plasma warmed, and thrombin reagent added typically human or bovine thrombin.
4. Incubate at 37°C.
5. Clot detection is performed by electro-mechanical or photo-optical methods.

Benefits: Quick and easy to perform. No special steps needed. Recognised by multiple specialities and hospitals.

Limitations: Traumatic venepuncture can lead to sample clotting. Does not give diagnosis. Affected by multiple conditions.

Prolongation: UFH (contamination), dabigatran use, fibrinogen deficiency (quantitative and qualitative), paraproteinaemia, amyloidosis, raised D-dimer.

Reduced by: Fibrinogen treatment or reactive causes of hyperfibrinogenaemia, though can also inversely prolong the TT in high doses.

Correction:

Heparin contamination: Corrects with protamine and toluidine blue. Prolonged Reptilase time also.

Fibrinogen deficiency: Corrects with normal plasma and not protamine or toluidine blue.

Dysfibrinogenaemia: Corrects with protamine and mostly with normal plasma addition. Check a Clauss fibrinogen assay in this scenario.

Further reading:

https://practical-haemostasis.com/Screening%20Tests/thrombin_time.html

Fibrinogen Assay

Introduction: The standard fibrinogen assay as part of the coagulation screen is a functional-based assay measuring fibrinogen activity. When low it may be appropriate to also measure fibrinogen levels, via a fibrinogen antigen assay.

What is measured: Fibrinogen quantity or function based on the assay.

Types: Clauss and PT derived: Functional assay (Fibrinogen activity).

Immunological or Clot weight: Quantitative assay (Fibrinogen antigen).

Normal range: Normal fibrinogen levels range from 1.5–4 g/L.

How to perform: (Clauss method)

1. Blood collected in blue top sodium citrate to line of tube for appropriate dilution for calcium chelation.
2. Sample centrifuged to collect plasma from red cells, platelets and mononuclear cells.
3. Plasma diluted with buffer and warmed to 37°C.
4. High concentration of thrombin is added which cleaves soluble fibrinogen to generate an insoluble fibrin clot that stabilises the platelet plug and initiates clot formation.
5. Time for clot to form is measured generally via optical density.
6. This time is plotted against a standard distribution curve which correlates with fibrinogen concentration.
7. The time is inversely proportional to the concentration of fibrinogen.

Benefits: WHO standardised test, most labs familiar with, various assays for FGN analysis.

Limitations: Traumatic venepuncture can lead to sample clotting. Acute phase protein which is affected in various disease states.

Reduced by: Congenital fibrinogen disorders which are rare, massive transfusion, DIC, liver disease, thrombolysis, neonatal apparent dysfibrinogenaemia due to altered sialylation.

Increased by: Female sex, malignancy, sepsis or other acute phase syndromes, old age.

Isolated reduced FGN: Perform immunological or clot weight assay for differential of hypo or dysfibrinogenaemia.

Reduced FGN and prolonged APTT and PT: Suggests hypofibrinogaenemia but rule out DIC.

Phrases for the essay: The Clauss fibrinogen assay is standardised by WHO calibration of plasma samples to produce the concentration curve.

Further reading:

https://practical-haemostasis.com/Screening%20Tests/fibrinogen.html

D-Dimer

Introduction: The D-dimer test is an analysis of the breakdown products of cross-linked fibrin molecules acting as an indicator of new VTE, although it can be raised in various other disease or physiological states without thrombosis.

What it measures: The action of plasmin on cross linked fibrin molecule. Assays can be quantitative, qualitative or both.

Types: Over 30 different assays for measuring a D-dimer, many focusing on the recognition of a specific epitope related to cross linked D-dimer molecules. For that reason, I will not describe how to do one given the wide range of ways to perform based on the different reagents and assays.

ELISA: Direct antibodies specific for D-dimer.

Latex agglutination immunoassay: Uses bispecific monoclonal antibodies.

Whole blood agglutination: Uses bispecific monoclonal antibodies.

Normal range: Varies based on assay used and lab ranges. Generally, < 500 ng/mL excludes VTE.

Benefits: Quick and easy to perform, less invasive and expensive than imaging for VTE i.e., CTPA or USS, used in VTE recurrence risk.

Limitations: Not specific, good screening tool but better for ruling out of VTE if clinical pre-test probability is low to moderate and D-dimer -ve (i.e. -ve predictive value), quantitative methods not standardised, assay variability across lab may give different reference ranges.

Reduced by: When normal can be used to rule out VTE in selected patients.

Increased by: VTE, acute phase i.e., pregnancy or trauma, old age, CKD, CCF.

Further reading:
https://practical-haemostasis.com/Fibrinolysis/d_dimers.html

Anti-Xa

Introduction: The anti-Xa activity assay is used to assess either the response (clearance or dosing) of patients on DOACS which inhibit anti-Xa or LMWH and UFH which work by inhibiting factor Xa and factor IIa. The anti-Xa assay for each DOACS is different and needs to be calibrated for each in the lab and cannot be transferred among different DOACS. Also used in children and high-risk patients for bleeding on treatment dose anticoagulation which inhibit Xa i.e., pregnancy.

What it measures: Measures peak or trough level of Xa inhibition based on anti-coagulant used. Can also measure DOACS level as well as anti-Xa but this requires specialist lab normally.

How to perform:

1. Blood collected in blue top sodium citrate to line of tube for appropriate dilution for calcium chelation. Document the medication the patient is on for the lab to run the correct assay.
2. Sample centrifuged to collect plasma from red cells, platelets and mononuclear cells.
3. A known amount of excess factor Xa is added to a set volume of the patient plasma.
4. Incubate at 37°C.
5. Complex formation occurs between drug in plasma and Xa added.
6. Set amount of chromogenic substrate added which binds to the residual/left over excess Xa not bound to drug in plasma.
7. Wavelength of light omitted which is measured by optical density.
8. Plotted along standardised curve of optical densities which correlate to drug concentration.
9. Each optical density is specific to the standardised curve of the drug being assessed. Clotting based assay can be performed instead which is an APTT based factor assay on remaining factor Xa rather than chromogenic.

Normal range: <u>Peak level</u>: 2–4 hours after dose 0.3–0.7 IU/ml though this varies according to the type of heparin or DOACS used, the dosing schedule and the relative Xa/IIa activity.

Benefits: Specific indication and can guide treatment decisions. Way of monitoring DOACS response in those without real impairment or extremes of weight compared to PT/APTT. Many labs have replaced APTTR with anti-Xa for monitoring of UFH infusions as more accurate.

Limitations: Time consuming. Trained staff and lab not always available. Relies on timing of blood taking and understanding of test. Often other medical specialities may request the wrong test.

Reduced by: Inadequate dosing, large body weight, increased clearance or dialysis.

Increased by: Overdose, low body weight, AKI or CKD causing reduced elimination.

Further reading:

https://practical-haemostasis.com/Miscellaneous/anti_xa_assays.html

Special Coagulation Tests

Mixing Study

Introduction: Mixing studies can be used in a prolonged APTT to assess the likely cause of the prolongation when using lupus sensitive reagents. Many labs have replaced them with factor assays and lupus anticoagulant screen in order to assess for a factor deficiency with a significant bleeding risk quicker.

What it measures: Either an inhibitor prolonging the assay is present or a true factor deficiency is present. Inhibitors can be drugs such as LMWH or DOACS, against a specific factor such as factor VIII inhibitor or non-specific such as lupus anticoagulant.

How to perform:
1. Ensure no anticoagulants have been given for 24–48 hours.
2. Blood collected in blue top sodium citrate to line of tube for appropriate dilution for calcium chelation.
3. Sample centrifuged to collect plasma from red cells, platelets and mononuclear cells.
4. APTT performed to confirm isolated prolongation.
5. Patient plasma mixed with normal reagent plasma in equal parts or can be in dilutions for more sensitivity in mild prolongation.
6. Time to clot formation performed as per APTT methodology. Can be immediate or incubated test depending on lab protocol.

Results interpretation:
No correction immediately: Immediate inhibitor.
No correction after incubation: Time-dependent inhibitor i.e., APTT becomes more prolonged over time.
Full correction: Time-dependent inhibitor or more likely a significant factor deficiency.

Benefits: Can rule out majority of factor deficiencies if it doesn't correct fully. Good screening prior to factor assays or inhibitor screen. Helps guide treatment in uncertain scenarios i.e., surgery.

Limitations: Multiple factor deficiencies may not correct and be an inhibitor. High haematocrit or underfilled tube. Anticoagulation effects. Not automated test and often needs to be directed by haem reg as referring speciality may struggle with result interpretation.

Factor Assays

Introduction: A factor assay is performed when there is prolongation of a screening coagulation test and there is correction upon 50:50 mixing study with normal test plasma. The 1-stage assay is either APTT or PT based. For the purposes of this assume we are performing a 1-stage APTT factor VIII assay.

What it measures: Any factor. Measures series of dilutions of the time taken to clot from the patient plasma and graph plotted to assess the percentage factor deficiency and severity based on known factor levels and times to clot from a reference plasma.

How to perform:
1. Ensure no anticoagulants have been given for 24–48 hours.
2. Blood collected in blue top sodium citrate to line of tube for appropriate dilution for calcium chelation.
3. Perform an APTT (see above) using factor VIII deficient plasma and reference plasma sample at relevant dilution with buffered saline. i.e., 50:50 = 1:2. 10:90 = 1:10 etc.
4. At least 3 dilutions should be performed as a minimum and APTT on each dilution.
5. Perform an APTT on just the reference/reagent plasma at various dilutions by buffering in normal saline. These should match the test plasma.
6. Each dilution for patient and reference plasma is plotted on a graph with clotting time on the Y axis and dilution on the X.
7. Check whether the lines are parallel. Non-parallelism suggests presence of an inhibitor or may be seen where factor deficiency is severe i.e., < 0.01 IU/ml. The clotting factor to which the inhibitor is directed will appear equally deficient at all dilutions.
8. Plot the lines at a said dilution to intersect the reference and patient plasma and then interpret the factor level from the known reference plasma in relation to the patient sample. Don't forget to correct for the concentration of factor in the reference plasma. i.e., if 90% multiply the final factor level by 0.9 to get true value. This will be on the reference plasma information sheet.

Results interpretation: Factor VIII levels diagnostic of disease phenotype below.
Mild haemophilia: 0.05–0.45 IU/ml.
Moderate haemophilia: 0.01–0.05 IU/ml.
Severe haemophilia: < 0.01 IU/ml.

Benefits: Quantifies factors and gives diagnosis. Robust test. Reference plasma for standardisation. Can be used for monitoring treatment response in haemophilia.

Limitations: User to do test however now often automated. Skewed by inhibitors. Specialist haemostasis lab needed. Often time consuming. Needs haematology specialist input. Doesn't always rule out VWD. Can be affected by acute state i.e., infection.

Further reading:
https://practical-haemostasis.com/Factor%20Assays/1_stage_aptt_factor_assay.html

Bethesda

Introduction: The Bethesda assay looks at isolating an inhibitor against factor VIII rather than a phospholipid inhibitor such as lupus anticoagulant. Performed and suspected when a prolonged clotting test does not correct on mixing, in congenital haemophilia A patients with suspected inhibitor development or when acquired haemophilia A is suspected.

What it measures: Quantifies the inhibitor against factor VIII. Measured in Bethesda units (BU). 1 BU is the ability of the inhibitor to neutralise 1 unit of factor VIII by 50% after 2 hours incubation. Factor VIII inhibitors are time dependent.

How to perform:

1. Ensure no anticoagulants have been given for 24–48 hours.
2. Blood collected in blue top sodium citrate to line of tube for appropriate dilution for calcium chelation.
3. Sample centrifuged to collect plasma from red cells, platelets and mononuclear cells.
4. Diluted patient plasma and pooled normal plasma are mixed at 1:1 ratio and then several dilutions made.
5. Mix buffer and the pooled normal plasma at 1:1 ratio as well and several dilutions made as control.
6. Incubate both at 37°C for 2 hours.
7. Measure residual factor VIII activity by 1-stage APTT.
8. Plot on graph and derive the Bethesda units from known reference range plotted on the graph.
9. Multiply by the dilution. I.e., if 2 BU in the 1:10 dilution then 20 BU in total.

Nijmegen modification: Normal plasma is buffered and in the control factor VIII deficient plasma is used to protect against changes in pH which can affect the factor VIII in the patient sample and inactivate it making the test less reliable. It is primarily done when a low titre BU is detected as this may be a false +ve. In Nijmegen modification a false +ve will show no inhibitor present and the false +ve is due to an inactivation of factor VIII via pH changes.

Results interpretation: As above for factor VIII reference ranges.

Straight line: A type 1 inhibitor/alloantibody in haemophilia A patients on treatment.

Curved line: A type 2 inhibitor, suggesting autoantibody often seen in acquired haemophilia A.

Benefits: Can distinguish different type of inhibitor and can monitor those on treatment.

Limitation: Fluctuations in pH and temperature can affect factor VIII stability. Small inhibitors not always able to detect. Time consuming with specialist lab needed. Can be tough to quantify inhibitor in those taking factor VIII concentrate.

Further reading:

https://practical-haemostasis.com/Inhibitor%20Assays/inhibitor_assays.html

Von Willebrand Tests

Introduction: There are multiple tests of VWF used to diagnose and distinguish between the various subtype of VWD.

What it measures: Often normal FBC, platelet count, APTT, PT and FGN unless significant reduction factor VIII. Often a VWF screen is performed, and then further tests as needed to characterise the VWD subtype. Below is what each test measures.

VWD initial screen:

VWF:Ag: The only quantitative assessment of VWF. Immunoturbidimetric has generally replaced ELISA.

VWF:CB: Qualitative assay that measures binding of VWF to Collagen. Indirect ELISA.

VWF:RCo: Qualitative assay looking at interaction between VWF and platelets, specifically A1 domain and GpIba receptor.

Factor VIII assay: See factor assay section.

VWF specialised tests:

HMW multimer analysis: Qualitative assay looking at concentrations of HMW multimer. Distinguishes between 2M and 2A.

VWF:Factor VIII binding study: Binding assay to look at VWF/factor VIII binding which will help identify type 2N.

Low dose RIPA: Qualitative analysis assessing platelet agglutination with VWF. Characterises type 2B VWD (where defect is in the part of VWF that binds platelet GpIb) or platelet-type VWD (sometimes referred to as pseudo VWD), where defect is in the platelet GpIba receptor.

Principle behind each test:

VWF:Ag: Immunoassay using latex beads coated in antibodies to VWF which bind VWF when plasma is passed over or mixed. Agglutination is measured by impedance of light which is proportional to VWF concentration.

VWF:CB: Indirect ELISA. Plasma passed through microplates coated in collagen. Wash to remove all not bound to collagen plates. Add solution of antibody with chromogenic substrate against VWF. Addition of enzyme to catalyse reaction and measure luminescence which correlates to binding activity.

VWF:RCo: RCo describes platelet agglutination using excess ristocetin and dilutions of plasma. Different methods and increasingly more automated. Ristocetin is used to induce change in VWF, whose activity is measured by platelet aggregation via light transmission aggregometry.

HMW multimer analysis: Gel based immune precipitation assay which can visualise the amount of multimers of different sizes as well as their pattern of triplet appearance.

VWF:Factor VIII binding study: Plasma from the patient is placed on microtiter plates with wells which capture VWF by antibody binding. Factor VIII is removed from VWF via washing with calcium chloride and a known amount of factor VIII is then added to the now VWF which is free from factor VIII. An antibody with a chromogenic substrate is added which hydrolyses the excess factor VIII and luminescence is measured. The intensity is proportional to the bound factor VIII to VWF. This assay is largely replaced by genetic analysis of factor VIII binding domains of VWF.

Low dose RIPA: Add limiting concentrations of ristocetin to undiluted platelet rich plasma. Agglutination at low concentrations of ristocetin resulting from gain-of-function is characteristic of type 2B or platelet-type VWD. Genetic testing is increasingly replacing RIPA testing. To distinguish between type 2b and platelet-type VWD mixing studies using platelets and plasma can be performed, although in practice this has largely been replaced by genetic analysis. Platelets are washed from the plasma and placed in normal plasma and the patient plasma has test normal platelets added. A RIPA is performed on each to observe agglutination and whether the defect is due to the plasma (type 2b) or platelets (pseudo VWD).

Mention molecular/genetic analysis as a method of testing in the exam!

Results interpretation:

VWF:Ag undetectable: Type 3.

Low Factor VIII or Factor VIII binding: Type 2N.

Low VWF:RCo or VWF:CB: Check RCo/Ag ratio. *Ratio > 0.7*: Type 1. *Ratio < 0.7*: Type 2 and then perform RIPA study to find sub-classification.

+ve low dose RIPA: Type 2B or platelet-type.

Normal RIPA: Type 2A or 2M so perform a multimer study or VWF:CB assay if not done already.

Loss of HMW multimers: Type 2A or Type 2B, confirmed with ratio of RCo:Ag and CB:Ag < 0.7.

All multimer sizes present: Type 2M, confirmed with ratio of RCo:Ag < 0.6; ratio of CB:Ag > 0.7.

Further reading:

https://onlinelibrary.wiley.com/doi/full/10.1111/bjh.13064

https://practical-haemostasis.com/Factor%20Assays/vwf/vwf_assays_introduction.html

Platelet Function Tests

Introduction: Platelet function tests are often performed on patients with a significant bleeding history who have normal APTT, PT and FGN and VWD screen. There are several tests looking at platelets number and function to aid in gaining a diagnosis.

What it measures: Disorder can either affect platelet number, function (due to granule issues) or receptor issues, as well as other associated coagulation disorder (Wiskott-Alrdich syndrome) or other non-haematological disorders (MYH9 disorders).

MPV: Useful for distinguishing between micro and macro-thrombocytopaenia disorders.

Film: Assessment of platelet morphology, granulation, size and colour. Also, neutrophil inclusions e.g., Döhle bodies seen in May-Hegglin.

LTA: Qualitative test using various agonists to assess platelet aggregation.

Impedance platelet aggregometry: Qualitative test on whole blood measuring platelet activation following addition of various agonist.

PFA-100/200: Whole blood Analysis of primary haemostatic function under high shear rate using apertures containing collagen and ADP or epinephrine. Sensitive to reduction in platelet number/function, quantitative and qualitative deficiencies VWF and low haematocrit.

Platelet nucleotide assay: Qualitative analysis of the 2 nucleotide pools within platelets to determine platelet granule disorders.

Flow cytometry: Analysis of platelet surface glycoproteins via specific antibodies with attached fluorochromes. Used for specific receptor abnormalities such as GpIIb/IIIa in Glanzmann's or GpIb in Bernard Soulier.

Principles behind each test: Stop all medications which affect platelets 7–10 days before tests and ideally done on site of testing so blood can reach the lab for testing ideally within 30–60 from draw.

LTA: Platelet rich and platelet poor plasma is collected via centrifugation and is incubated at 37°C and stirred. Ideally platelet count should be between $100–600 \times 10^9/L$ in PRP. Upon addition of various agonists, the platelets will aggregate or not depending on the disorder. The aggregation alters light transmission detected via the photocell and is recorded for each agonist to determine specific defects based on the aggregation wave produced. Controls for light transmission is performed on PRP and PPP.

PFA-100/200: Citrated blood is aspirated through disposable cartridges which have multiple open apertures. The apertures are coated with agonists based on the cartridge selected i.e., aspirin or collagen. Cartridges are coated with collagen, to reflect the subendothelium, together with either ADP or epinephrine as agonist. Upon interaction with the aspirated blood, platelets will be triggered or not to aggregate with the agonists. This causes the aperture to close over or remain open based on the reaction and can be measured. Ensure platelet count $> 100 \times 10^9/L$, not on aspirin, normal haematocrit and performed within 4 hours of blood collection.

<u>Platelet nucleotide assay</u>: Looks at the nucleotide pools of platelets which are either metabolically active (alpha granules) or inactive (dark granules). These pools have different ATP to ADP concentrations in various disorders, such as storage pool disorders (Hermansky-Pudlak syndrome. A classic exam question refers to this syndrome in a bleeding patient from Puerto Rico). The release of ATP from platelets is measured via a luciferin buffer which creates light upon ATP release and this is measured via a lumi-aggregometer.

<u>Flow cytometry</u>: Antibodies can be used which stain and recognise specific glycoproteins i.e., CD41 and GpIIb. Various flow patterns exist for various disorders based on these antibodies.

Results interpretation: For specific information see platelet function disorders section.

Further reading:

https://practical-haemostasis.com/Platelets/platelet_function_testing_introduction.html

https://onlinelibrary.wiley.com/doi/10.1111/bjh.17690

Bleeding Disorders

Haemophilia A

Introduction: A rare X-Linked bleeding disorder leading to an inability to produce sufficient factor VIII which leads to an increased risk of traumatic or spontaneous bleeding.

Epidemiology: 25:100,000 males. Accounts for 80% of haemophilia cases. Varying severity based on factor VIII level. Carrier females likely have a milder factor VIII deficiency, usually in mild range unless extreme lyonization or where both X chromosomes affected, which is rare.

Age of diagnosis: At any age but commonly in babies or when toddlers start to crawl or move more when no family history. Easier to diagnose if family history. Average age of first joint bleed in severe disease is 1–2 years old but should be on prophylaxis by then as aim is to avoid this.

Signs/symptoms: Bleeding at unusual sites such as joints, organs or muscles, easy bruising, spontaneous bleeding, uncontrolled bleeding.

Diagnosis:
- Isolated prolonged APTT.
- Use of bleeding assessment tool, family and clinical history as screening.
- Factor VIII assay shows level of < 0.45 IU/ml for diagnosis.

Pathophysiology: X-linked disorder due to mutation in the factor VIII gene.

Staging: Based on factor level.

Mild: 0.05–0.45 IU/ml.

Moderate: 0.1–0.5 IU/ml.

Severe: < 0.01 IU/ml.

Tx at diagnosis? Depends on severity. Treatment was previously based on when to initiate prophylaxis, especially in severe disease. Lifelong prophylaxis recommended and modern practice is now to start primary prophylaxis at diagnosis to prevent joint or severe bleeds in severe disease. Also initiated in moderate disease with factor level between 1–3%. Goal is to prevent bleeds and have a "normal" or non-bleeding phenotype.

Other important work up: Exclude other bleeding disorders such as type 2N VWD or acquired haemophilia A. Drug history and use of BAT, CVC line, virology testing at baseline i, e. HIV, hepatitis and other blood borne viruses which is relevant if known haemophilia patient who has received plasma derived products but not relevant for new diagnosis as products now recombinant.

First line tx: Choice of product discussed with patient. Recombinant now used over plasma derived. Extended half-life products are also available. Multiple agents WHO recommended to choose from. Use of a bypassing agent used to be recommended in those who develop and inhibitor against a factor concentrate that neutralises its efficacy, but practice now is to use the bispecific antibody Emicizumab.

Mild disease: DDAVP or TXA in bleeding or pre-procedure. May need factor concentrate if severe bleeding or high bleeding risk procedure.

Dosing: Generally, 20–40 units/kg of body weight. Half-life 8–12 hours.

Weight multiplied by desired factor level multiplied by 0.5 = IU of factor needed.

Regimes: Can be high (25–40 IU/kg 2 days), intermediate (15–25 IU/kg 3 days/week) or low dose (10–15 IU/kg 2–3 days/week).

The aim is to maintain a non-bleeding phenotype. Dosing intervals based on factor response and bleeding phenotype.

Specific scenarios target levels (IU/ml): Acute bleeds require immediate (within 2 hours) and ongoing treatment with factor replacement to stop bleeding and maintain haemostasis.

Joint bleed: > 0.5 IU/ml.

Muscle bleed: > 0.4 IU/ml.

Deep muscle or neurovascular injury: > 0.8 IU/ml.

ICB, GI or neck: > 0.8 IU/ml.

Minor op: *Pre*: > 0.5 IU/ml. *Post*: > 0.3 IU/ml.

Major op: *Pre*: > 0.8 IU/ml. *Post*: > 0.6 IU/ml.

Second/third line tx:

Emicizumab: Bispecific monoclonal antibody. Licensed in severe disease with or without inhibitors or in those not suitable or intolerant of factor replacement, but in reality, it is used first line in many patients with and without inhibitors.

Recombinant VIIa or bypassing agent: if Emicizumab contraindicated or not tolerated.

Inhibitor treatment: Immune tolerance induction once titre < 10 Bethesda Units. Regime and dosing depend on the titre. Agents such as FEIBA used which is bypassing agent can be used for bleeds, but high dose FVIII needed for immunotolerance +/- immunosuppressant therapy. Usually achieve tolerance by 1 year.

Prognosis: Joint or intracranial bleeds associated with worse prognosis and QOL.

High risk for inhibitor development: Large gene mutations, African ethnicity, family history, early exposure age, during 10–50 exposure days of treatment or intense first exposure i.e., infusion of factor VIII due to severe life-threatening bleed.

Important side effects: Thrombosis risk, risk of blood borne viruses from plasma derived products (though very low), inhibitor development, CVC line infection or thrombosis.

Monitoring: Maintain trough factor levels > 0.01 IU/ml at all times, ideally 0.3 IU/ml or until normal bleeding phenotype. Peak monitoring done 15–30 mins after dose. Trough level taken before the next dose is given.

Trials to quote: <u>ESPRIT trial</u>: Benefits of primary and secondary prophylaxis in reducing significant joint disease in severe haemophilia A.

Supportive care: Physiotherapy for hemarthrosis, clinical psychologist, CNS for family and patient support, pain team.

Other considerations: MRI or USS for assessing joint bleeds rather than CT or X-ray. Pharmacokinetics studies. Treatment in recognised tertiary haemophilia centre or transfer to once stable. **PRICE** for joints: **P**rotect, **R**aise, **I**ce, **C**ompress, **E**levate.

Inhibitor screening regularly until greater than 150 Exposure days. Register with national haemophilia database. Patient alert card.

Guidelines:

https://onlinelibrary.wiley.com/doi/10.1111/bjh.16704

https://haemophilia.org.uk/wp-content/uploads/pdf/WFH-Guidelines-for-the-Management-of-Hemophilia-3rd-edition.pdf

Haemophilia B

Introduction: A rare X-Linked bleeding disorder leading to an inability to produce sufficient factor IX which leads to an increased risk of traumatic or spontaneous bleeding.

Epidemiology: 5:100,000 males, accounts for 20% of haemophilia cases. Varying severity based on factor IX level. Females often not affected unless both X chromosomes affected as mentioned above.

Age of onset: Commonly in babies or toddlers when start to crawl if no family history though often made through family history screening at birth. Average age of first joint bleed in severe disease is 1–2 years old.

Signs/symptoms: Bleeding at unusual sites such as joints, organs or muscles, easy bruising, spontaneous bleeding, uncontrolled bleeding.

Diagnosis:
- Isolated prolonged APTT.
- Use of bleeding assessment tool, family and clinical history as screening.
- Factor IX assay shows level of < 0.40 IU/ml for diagnosis.

Pathophysiology: X-linked disorder due to mutation in the factor IX gene.

Staging: Based on factor level.

Mild: 0.05–0.45 IU/ml.

Moderate: 0.01–0.05 IU/ml.

Severe: < 0.01 IU/ml.

Tx at diagnosis? As above.

Other important work up: As above.

First line tx: Recommended to use concentrate containing only factor IX, rather than multiple factor such as PCC. Extended half-life products available if increasing treatment burden or other complications.

Regimes: Can be high (40–60 IU/kg 2 days/week), intermediate (20–40 IU/kg 2 days/week) or low dose (10–15 IU/kg 2 days/week).

Specific scenarios target levels (IU/ml): Acute bleeds require immediate (within 2 hours) and ongoing treatment with factor replacement to stop bleeding and maintain haemostasis.

Joint bleed: > 0.5 IU/ml.

Muscle bleed: > 0.4 IU/ml.

Deep muscle or neurovascular injury: > 0.6 IU/ml.

ICB, GI or neck: > 0.6 IU/ml.

Minor op: *Pre*: > 0.5 IU/ml. *Post*: > 0.3 IU/ml.

Major op: *Pre*: > 0.6 IU/ml. *Post*: > 0.4 IU/ml.

Second/third line tx: Recombinant factor VIIa if anaphylaxis to factor IX concentrate or inhibitor acquisition rather than PCC initially.

Inhibitor treatment: Immune tolerance induction once titre < 10 Bethesda units. Regime and dosing depend on the titre. Careful consideration in haemophilia B as low success rate (25%) and chance of anaphylaxis or CKD in the form of nephrotic syndrome. If needed, consider concomitant use of immunosuppressive drugs to improve success rate.

Prognosis: Joint or intracranial bleeds associated with worse prognosis and QOL.

High risk for inhibitor development: Large gene mutations, high dose at initial exposure (median time 11 exposure days), minimal other data on risk factors compared to haemophilia A.

Important side effects: Inhibitors associated with life threatening allergic reaction to factor concentrate. If anaphylaxis should prompt inhibitor screening. Thrombotic risk with high dose of factor concentrates.

Monitoring: Maintain trough factor levels > 0.01 IU/ml at all times, ideally > 0.03 IU/ml or until normal bleeding phenotype. Peak monitoring done 15–30 mins after dose. Trough level done before the next dose is given.

Supportive care: Physiotherapy for hemarthrosis, clinical psychologist, CNS for family and patient support, pain team.

Other considerations: MRI or USS for assessing joint bleeds rather than CT or X-ray. Pharmacokinetic studies. Treatment in recognised tertiary haemophilia centre or transfer to once stable. **PRICE** for joints: **P**rotect, **R**aise, **I**ce, **C**ompress, **E**levate. Inhibitor screening regularly until greater than 150 exposure days. Register with national haemophilia database. Patient alert card.

Guidelines:

https://onlinelibrary.wiley.com/doi/10.1111/bjh.16704

https://haemophilia.org.uk/wp-content/uploads/pdf/WFH-Guidelines-for-the-Management-of-Hemophilia-3rd-edition.pdf

Von Willebrand Disease

Introduction: Inherited bleeding disorder with numerous subtypes characterised by quantitative or qualitative deficiency in VWF.

Epidemiology: Most common inherited bleeding disorder. Up to 1% of population, autosomal inheritance pattern although more commonly diagnosed in females due to nature of haemostatic challenges such as menstruation and pregnancy.

Signs/symptoms: Spontaneous, large volume or excessive bleeding. Predominantly mucocutaneous bleeding. Common bleeding includes menorrhagia, bruising, post-partum or surgery, epistaxis, post-procedure, cutaneous bleeding, excessive bleeding from minor wounds such as shaving. Often normal APTT, always normal PT.

Diagnosis: VWF: Ag, factor VIII assay and VWF platelet binding activity (VWF: RCo or VWF: GpIb binding) used as screening.

- Bleeding assessment tool, family and clinical history as screening.
- VWF < 0.3 IU/ml sufficient for diagnosis.
- 0.3–0.5 IU/ml = low VWF but not diagnostic of VWD as per UK guidelines.

Other investigations such as RIPA, multimer analysis or VWF: CB used in secondary classification.

Pathophysiology: VWF is a large glycoprotein with multimers in varying molecular sizes. It is synthesised in bone marrow megakaryocytes, platelets and vascular endothelial cells. VWF has 2 main functions: Carries factor VIII and adheres to platelets and collagen on endothelial wall following trauma. VWF gene on chromosome 12 has 52 exons and the protein has multiple domains which correlate with some VWD subtypes due to either deficient or dysfunctional VWF protein or loss of HMW multimers of VWF. Autosomal dominant pattern in all subtypes except type 2N and 3, which are recessive.

Classification: See VWD assays for classification.

Tx at diagnosis? Depends on subtype, clinical history and clinical context.

Other important work up: Family history, rule out Acquired Von Willebrand Syndrome i.e., Consider screen for ET, LPD, MM or amyloidosis, valvular disease. DDAVP trial and genetic testing may clarify diagnosis. Blood borne viruses at baseline prior to plasma components.

First line tx: Divided into non-concentrate and concentrate therapies. Concentrate used in severe disease or those not responding to DDAVP.

Non-concentrate therapies:

DDAVP: IV, SC or Intranasal. Contraindicated in children < 2, relatively contraindicated in type 2b VWD. Ineffective in more severe type 1, type 3 and many type 2. Avoid when history of cardiovascular disease. Lack of consensus on upper age cut off, UK guidelines state 60 years. Limit fluid intake 24 hours after. Works by releasing factor VIII and VWF from endothelial stores.

TXA: IV, PO, topical or mouthwash in combination with DDAVP or in isolation for minor bleeding or pre-procedure.

Concentrate therapies:

High purity: Contains VWF only. Examples include Wilfacto (plasma derived) or Veyvondi (recombinant). Typically, 1 IU/Kg of VWF raises circulating VWF levels by 0.02 IU/ml. Should now be using recombinant VWF to prevent/treat bleeding episodes, not yet licensed in children or for prophylaxis. Used in long term prophylaxis or to prevent or treat bleed +/- factor VIII concentrate.

Intermediate purity: Contains VWF and factor VIII i.e., Voncento. Recommended in acute bleeding episodes.

Prophylaxis: Done in all VWD subtypes with or prone to recurrent bleeding episodes.

Specific scenarios:

Minor op: Keep VWF and FVIII > 0.5 IU/ml. May be achieved with DDAVP and TXA only.

Major op: Maintain FVIII > 0.5 IU/ml, VWF:RCo > 0.5 IU/ml at least 3 days post-op.

Pregnancy: *Type 1*: Manage as normal if VWF:RCo > 0.5 IU/ml.

Epidural: Avoid in type 2, 3 or if VWF:RCo not normalised in type 1. Keep VWF:RCo > 0.5 IU/ml for 6 hours after epidural removal.

Important side effects:

DDAVP: Flushing, hypotension and hyponatraemia.

Concentrates: Angioedema, thrombosis and inhibitor development.

Monitoring:

DDAVP: Peak response at 30–60 mins and check for rapid fall at 4–6 hours. > 0.3 IU/ml considered responsive.

Concentrates: Depends on scenario. In acute bleeding or surgery, at least twice a day to guide dosing.

Inhibitors: Consider if anaphylaxis reaction to concentrate. Use recombinant factor VIII, recombinant VIIIa, platelets or TXA if inhibitor.

Trials to quote: VWD international prophylaxis study: Role or prophylaxis in severe unresponsive VWD.

Other considerations: Do not wait until bleeding symptoms in children with family history. Test after 6 months to avoid false -ve. Importance of adjunctive therapy e.g., hormonal contraception to control gynaecological bleeding. Managed in haemophilia centre and specialist obstetric unit. Patient alert card.

Guidelines:

https://onlinelibrary.wiley.com/doi/full/10.1111/bjh.13064

https://ashpublications.org/bloodadvances/article/5/1/301/474884/ASH-ISTH-NHF-WFH-2021-guidelines-on-the-management

Acquired Haemophilia A

Introduction: Rare acquired bleeding disorder due to inhibitor/antibody development against factor VIII associated with several conditions.

Epidemiology: 1:1,000,000 per year. Median age of onset 75. Female predominance.

Signs/symptoms: May be associated with autoimmune disorders such as SLE or RA, pregnancy/postpartum or malignancy. Commonly, no associated factor is found. Presents with new onset bleeding, severe in 30%, note distinctive bleeding pattern from congenital haemophilia A with bleeding sites such as muscle, GU, GI, retroperitoneal. Joint bleeding rare.

Diagnosis: The immediate mixing study corrects and then becomes abnormal when incubated over time as they are often time and temperature dependent inhibitors. Important to exclude LA, especially if underlying autoimmune disease.

- Isolated prolonged APTT.
- Nonlinear/parallel factor VIII assay suggests inhibitor or a diagnosis of acquired haemophilia A.
- Positive Bethesda assay.

Tx at diagnosis? Patients generally present with bleeding so the answer is almost always yes.

Other important work up: Look for underlying cause, BAT, drug history, family history.

First line tx: Goals are to manage/prevent bleeding, eradicate inhibitor and manage symptoms or side effects of bleeding/treatment.

<u>Supportive care</u>: Avoid invasive procedures, minimise venepuncture and phlebotomy, analgesia for painful muscle bleeds.

<u>Treating bleeding</u>: Treat with bypassing agent i.e., FEIBA or recombinant factor VIIIa, though increasing use of Emicizumab reduces requirement for bypassing agent. TXA in mucosal bleeding. IVIG licensed in life or limb threatening bleeding after failed first line therapy but not in inhibitor eradication.

<u>Inhibitor eradication</u>: Start immunosuppression at diagnosis. Typically, 1 mg/kg of prednisolone daily +/- cyclophosphamide 1–2 mg/day.

Rituximab can be used if above contraindicated but response not as good. Usually used in second line treatment. If no response after 1 month switch to second line therapy as above or considered MMF, ciclosporin or cytotoxic. Evidence not strong enough to recommend immune tolerance regime with factor VIII and immunosuppression.

Important side effects: Thrombotic risk with bypassing agent increased. TXA as mentioned above. Neutropaenia, anaemia, infection, thrombocytopaenia in immunosuppression. Steroid side effects as previously mentioned.

Monitoring: Monthly follow up for first 6 months checking factor VIII level and inhibitor screen. If factor VIII normal assess thrombotic risk.

Prognosis: Mortality rates based on PS, treatment and severity. 5% mortality from bleeding. 10% for complications of immunosuppression.

Trials to quote: EACH2: Bypassing agents best at achieving haemostasis.

UKHCDO: Relapse occurs in 20% of patients.

Other considerations: Treat in haemophilia centre with experience in management. Register with national haemophilia database. Patient alert card. Coagulation screen and factor VIII level prior to procedures and close liaison with haematology pre, peri and post-operatively.

Guidelines:

https://onlinelibrary.wiley.com/doi/full/10.1111/bjh.12463

Acquired Von Willebrand Syndrome

Introduction: Rare acquired bleeding disorder associated with various conditions leading to functional defects in VWF. These commonly occur due to antibody mediated dysfunction, VWF adsorption onto the cell of origin driving the defect (as in ET) or mechanical shear stresses causing VWF proteolysis.

Epidemiology: Few cases to give true incidence but rare. Most common underlying disorders are myeloma/MGUS, LPD, MPN (especially ET), aortic stenosis (Heyde's syndrome) or following assisted ventricular device insertion. Solid organ malignancy but less commonly.

Signs/symptoms: New bleeding history, previously no bleeding history following surgery or pregnancy etc, new associated condition, no family history, improved bleeding phenotype following treatment of underlying disorder, normal molecular testing.

Diagnosis: Consider if there is a new bleeding history with associated disorder and associated VWF tests i.e., reduced VWF:Ag or RCo, FVIII:C, loss of HMW. Testing for VWF binding antibodies or inhibitor may be +ve in mixing studies done on VWF:Ag or RCo. If diagnosis in question, consider molecular testing to rule out inherited VWD which is more typical as difficult to always isolate and identify antibodies.

Pathophysiology: Multiple pathways as mentioned above. Neutralising antibodies against any binding site of VWF i.e., to collagen or platelets. Increased clearance of VWF due to coating or antibody binding. Decreased synthesis of VWF or proteolytic breakdown of HMW multimers.

Tx at diagnosis? Yes, unless asymptomatic but patients rarely diagnosed when asymptomatic.

Other important work up: Look for associated condition is the most important thing as treatment of it improves chances of resolution.

First line tx: Goals are to manage/prevent bleeding and reduce/eradicate inhibitor often by treating underlying cause to completed remission.

Treating bleeding: IVIG in IgG paraproteinaemia. TXA in all.

Use of VWF concentrates in acute or major bleeding and may need higher doses and greater dose frequency. Bypassing agents such as recombinant factor VIIa in those who develop alloantibodies in addition to autoantibodies.

Inhibitor eradication: Depends on underlying cause. In essence, treat underlying cause for best chance at definitive treatment.

Important side effects: As mentioned above for VWD.

Monitoring: No specific guidance but advisable to follow acquired haemophilia A guidance in terms of how and when to monitor.

Guidelines:
https://ashpublications.org/blood/article/117/25/6777/24352/How-I-treat-the-acquired-von-Willebrand-syndrome
https://onlinelibrary.wiley.com/doi/full/10.1111/bjh.13064

Hypo and Dysfibrinogenaemia

Introduction: Rare autosomal bleeding disorder leading to qualitative or quantitative FGN protein defects.

Epidemiology: 1:1,000,000 people affected as autosomal recessive inheritance. Incidence of autosomal dominant inheritance not known.

Signs/symptoms:

Hypo and afibrinogenemia: Excessive bleeding from surgery or trauma. Common sites include soft tissue, mucosal, cutaneous, GU, joint and menstrual. 5% ICB. Rare symptoms include splenic rupture or liver disease. Prolonged PT, and TT usually.

Dysfibrinogenaemia: 50% asymptomatic, can cause bleeding which is often mucosal, cutaneous, or post-surgery OR thrombosis in 20% especially in those where the mutation is near the thrombin-cleavage site, though FGN assays can't distinguish between clinical phenotypes.

Diagnosis: The way to distinguish between hypo and dysfibrinogenaemia also requires measuring fibrinogen level via an immunological or clot weight-based assay.

- Clinical history.
- Reduced FGN by Clauss assay often < 1.5 g/L in hypofibrinogenemia and 0.1–0.8 g/L in dysfibrinogenemia.
- Prolonged PT, and TT usually in both.

Pathophysiology: Affected genes include those responsible for FGN production which are *FGA*, *FGB* and *FGG*. The FGN disorder inherited often depends on the gene or genes affected which in turn affects the respective glycoprotein chain making up the FGN molecule. Dysfunctional FGN molecules lead to reduced platelet adhesion and aggregation and hence ineffective haemostasis initiation. Reduced FGN molecule production reduces the effectiveness of initial haemostasis due to inability to form a stable strong mesh with platelet adhesion.

Classification: See FGN assays for which assay to use. Can be either afibrinogenemia, hypofibrinogenemia or dysfibrinogenaemia.

Mild: >1 g/L.

Moderate: 0.1–1 g/L.

Severe: Undetectable and a discrepancy seen between function and antigen.

Tx at diagnosis? Not always, especially in mild/moderate forms if no bleeding or procedures planned.

Severe: Consider long term prophylaxis.

Other important work up: Family history and use of BAT, virology testing at baseline if previously received plasma products i.e., HIV, hepatitis and other blood borne viruses, rule out DIC.

First line tx:

Hypo and afibrinogenemia: Fibrinogen concentrate (Riastap) in severe bleeding or major surgery. TXA in minor bleeding. Dose based on target level minus the measured level and divided by 0.017 to give the mg/kg. Aim generally to keep FGN > 1 g/L at least. 4–6 g total dose rises serum FGN by 1–1.5 g/L. Pathogen reduced cryoprecipitate if FGN concentrate not available. Dose is 15–20 ml/kg.

Dysfibrinogenaemia: Fibrinogen concentrate (Riastap) in severe bleeding or major surgery. TXA in minor. Cryoprecipitate if no concentrate. Beware thrombotic complications if rapid rise in serum total FGN and VTE prophylaxis when haemostasis achieved.

Specific scenarios:

Prophylaxis: FGN < 0.1 g/L and severe bleeding history. FGN concentrate once a week to target trough FGN > 0.5 g/L.

Pregnancy: FGN < 0.5 g/L or previous complicated pregnancy. FGN concentrate twice a week to target trough FGN > 1 g/L.

Paeds: Typically, weekly prophylaxis with cryoprecipitate or FGN concentrate. Target trough FGN 0.5–1 g/L. May present with umbilical or ICB.

Dysfibrinogenaemia with no bleeding: TXA if needed. More importantly routine VTE prophylaxis should be given as required.

Important side effects: As previously mentioned for TXA. Thrombotic complications. Reactions or infection from cryoprecipitate.

Other considerations: Thromboprophylaxis in dysfibrinogenaemia with thrombotic tendency postpartum or procedure.

Guidelines:

https://onlinelibrary.wiley.com/doi/full/10.1111/bjh.13058

https://onlinelibrary.wiley.com/doi/full/10.1046/j.1365-2141.2003.04256.x

Platelet Function Disorders

Introduction: Umbrella term for several IPD which lead to abnormal platelet function and bleeding with or without thrombocytopaenia. They often have underlying molecular abnormalities and can have associated other conditions.

Incidence: 10% of bleeding disorders in national haemophilia database, over 50 different recognised disorders.

Signs/symptoms: Bleeding, bruising and petechial rash generally.

MYH-9 e.g., MHA: Cataracts, deafness, nephropathy, neutrophil inclusions.

WAS: Immunodeficiency, infections, LPD.

CHS: Albinism, immunodeficiency, HLH.

GPS: Myelofibrosis.

HPS: Albinism, immunodeficiency, albinism, granulomatous colitis, pulmonary fibrosis, from Puerto Rico.

Diagnosis: Diagnosis is made generally using several different tests following clinical history and normal APTT, PT, FGN and TT.

Morphology: Giant platelets, anisocytosis of platelets, grey platelets in granule disorders, Döhle bodies in neutrophils in MHA.

LTA: Series of agonists to activate platelets, certain disorders produce recognised aggregation curve pattern. Full agonist panel includes ADP, epinephrine, TXA2, collagen, ristocetin, arachidonic acid and PAR1. Important to perform on PRP. May not be possible if low platelet count. See below for most common IPD diagnostic patterns.

Flow cytometry: Antibodies against certain platelet receptors i.e., CD41 and CD61 in Glanzmann's and CD42a and b in BSS.

PDA100/200: Platelet function assay looking at high shear rates and activation with epinephrine, collagen, ADP or P2Y12.

Platelet nucleotide assay/Lumi-aggregometry: Done if LTA normal, diagnosis of storage pool disorders, looks at ADP:ATP ratio following agonist.

Classification: Based on MPV i.e., micro, normo or macrothrombocytic. Or classify based on aggregation response.

Glanzmann's: GpIIb/IIIa defect.

BSS: GpIb-IX-V defect.

Storage pool disorders: Alpha or delta granule defects.

MYH-9 and WAS: Structural cytoskeletal defects due to molecular abnormalities.

Secretion disorders: Defects in receptors for agonists.

Tx at diagnosis? Depends on bleeding phenotype but prophylactic may be needed if severe. Treat when bleeding.

Other important work up: BAT, assessment for other disease such as infection or albinisms which may point you to diagnosis, previous surgical history, drug history, genetic analysis should be done in all suspected of IPD.

First line tx: Local measures like TXA soaks or washes, oral or IV if needed. Platelet transfusion using HLA matched platelets. DDAVP in storage disorders. Recombinant factor VIIa if haemostasis not achieved. Consider BMT in severe disorders like WAS.

Other considerations: Register with national haemophilia database, counsellor, stop medications 7–10 days pre-test. Ideally sampling done on site where test takes place.

Guidelines:

https://onlinelibrary.wiley.com/doi/10.1111/bjh.17690

IPD pathological defect and the aggregation response expected to agonists in aggregation studies.

IPD	Pathological defect	ADP	Adrenaline	Collagen	Ristocetin	Arachidonic acid
BSS	GP-Ib-IX-V	Normal	Normal	Normal	Inhibited	Normal
Glanzmann thrombasthenia	GP-Ib-IIIa	Inhibited	Inhibited	Inhibited	Normal	Inhibited
MYH-9 like disorders	*MYH-9 gene*	Normal	Normal	Normal	Normal	Normal
Aspirin	COX-1 inhibitor and reduced TXA2 production	Initial aggregation only	Initial aggregation only	Inhibited	Normal	Inhibited
Clopidogrel	Glycoprotein IIb/IIIa inhibition	Inhibited	Normal	Variable inhibition	Normal	Normal
Storage pool disorders	Delta or alpha granule formation or release	Initial aggregation only	Initial aggregation only	Initial aggregation only	Variable inhibition	Normal
Type 2b VWD	Gain of function in VWF gene and increased binding via glycoprotein Ib	Normal	Normal	Normal	Inhibited but normal aggregation with low dose ristocetin	Normal

Thrombosis

Provoked and Unprovoked VTE

Introduction: Venous or arterial occlusion due to venous stasis, hypercoagulability or vascular injury which can be provoked or unprovoked.

Signs/symptoms: Hot, swollen, painful calf. New varicose veins with associated symptoms. Shortness of breath or haemoptysis, pleuritic chest pain, other local symptoms.

Diagnosis: D-dimer can be used to rule out DVT or PE with sensitivity of > 95%. Wells score for likelihood of VTE or PE. > 4 PE/DVT likely and should do an USS. If NAD but symptoms persist repeat in 1 week and consider treatment in that week if strong history for VTE provided low bleeding risk. CTPA unless pregnant then consider V/Q scan due to risk of radiation to mother's breast tissue. Consider CT Angio in proximal DVT as may need thrombolytic directed therapy from vascular team if extension into iliac vein.

Classification:

Provoked: Underlying cause or transient event within 3 months identified which led to VTE.

Recurrent: More than 1 VTE, which can be provoked or unprovoked but often leads to lifelong anticoagulation.

Proximal: DVT affecting veins above the knee, at the junction of the popliteal vein i.e., femoral, iliac or popliteal. Higher risk of embolising to become PE than distal.

Distal: A DVT affecting veins below the knee i.e., peroneal, posterior, anterior tibial, and muscular veins.

Risk factors: Major or minor provoking factors include surgery, pregnancy, delivery and postpartum, inherited thrombophilia, smoking, obesity, long haul flights, periods of immobility, cancer, age, heart failure, chronic inflammatory disorders, medications i.e., COCP.

Tx at diagnosis? Yes, with treatment dose anticoagulation unless significant bleeding risk outweighing benefit.

Other important work up: Search for provoking factors, family history, thrombophilia screen if indicated from family history, APS and antithrombin-III most important in affecting treatment decisions. Appropriate cancer screening based on sex, symptoms and age.

First line tx: Treatment dose anticoagulation. LMWH based on weight. Warfarin based on INR monitoring. Most would start DOACS now unless contraindication, not licensed or patient preference. Consider IVC filter in DVT with those who are unable to have treatment dose anticoagulation (intracranial bleed or severe thrombocytopaenia).

Provoked: 3 months minimum provided the provoking factor has gone. 6 months in cancer associated. DOACS first line either apixaban or rivaroxaban though dabigatran or edoxaban can be used also with 5 days of LMWH lead in. LMWH for 5 days also then warfarin if DOACS contraindicated.

Unprovoked: 3 months minimum but consider lifelong based on risk factor, proximity and investigate causes.

Proximal or PE: 3 months minimum or lifelong based on risk factors. Consider longer if extension to iliac vein or if multiple PE. DOACS first line.

Distal: 3 months. Consider longer if provoking factor still present.

Superficial: 6 weeks and reassess.

Recurrent: Lifelong therapy.

Specific scenarios:

Pregnancy: DOACS not licensed as crosses placenta. Warfarin embryopathy 6–12 weeks' gestation. DOACS contraindicated if breastfeeding, but warfarin safe.

Renal failure: Dose reduce LMWH and DOACS. DOACS contraindicated in CrCl < 15 ml/min though different thresholds exist across different DOACS.

Extremes of weight: Regular monitoring in < 50 kg and > 120 kg with anti-Xa levels or INR. DOACS not contraindicated but 30% lower or higher exposure in excess or reduced bodyweight respectively.

Cancer: Treat for 3–6 months and longer if cancer still active. LMWH previously shown to be most effective, although DOACS now being used more frequently provided bleeding risk assessed. Higher bleeding risk in mucosal tumours i.e., GI or bladder.

Important side effects: Assess bleeding risk with HAS-BLED score and plan for breaks or bridging during procedures.

Monitoring: INR used in Warfarin therapy. Anti-Xa-based assays can be used in specific situations in LMWH and DOACS. Consider USS at time of cessation of anticoagulant therapy as useful baseline in case future symptoms. Helps to distinguish post-thrombotic syndrome from new VTE.

Scoring:

Well's: Clinical prediction tool — risk of VTE or PE based on symptoms.

DASH: Risk of VTE recurrence based on D-dimer, age, gender and whether event was oestrogen provoked.

HERDOO2: Risk of discontinuation of anticoagulation in women based on D-dimer, age and post-thrombotic syndrome symptoms.

Khorana: Risk of VTE in cancer patients based on cancer type, BMI and FBC parameters.

Trials to quote:

ROCKET AF: Rivaroxaban vs warfarin in AF non-inferior and better intracranial bleeding rates.

ARISTOTLE: Apixaban vs Warfarin in stroke prevention in AF.

ENGAGE-AF: Edoxaban vs Warfarin in stroke prevention in AF.

RE-LY: Dabigatran vs Warfarin in stroke prevention in AF.

Guidelines:

https://www.nice.org.uk/guidance/ng158

https://www.aafp.org/pubs/afp/issues/2011/0201/p293.html#:~:text=Patients%20 with%20a%20VTE%20and,as%20the%20cancer%20is%20active

Thrombosis at Unusual Sites

Central Venous Sinus

Epidemiology: Affects young adults, female predominance. 4:1,000,000. Fairly rare.
Signs/symptoms: Headache, focal neurology, intracranial hypertension, cerebral infarction and oedema.
Diagnosis: MRI ideally but high-resolution CT or Angio if MRI not available.
Risk factors: Infection, MPN, leukaemia, asparaginase treatment, obesity, trauma, pregnancy or COCP often combined with factor V Leiden or other thrombophilia.
Tx at diagnosis? Yes, even if intracranial bleeding then continue anticoagulation.
First line tx: LMWH treatment dose for 7 days. Warfarin for 3 months minimum. UFH infusion considered if intracranial bleeding so can monitor and stop easily. Surgical decompression if brain stem herniation from raised ICP. DOACS can be considered after initial heparin treatment.

Retinal Vein Occlusion

Epidemiology: Associated with older age. 1:200 per year in over 65's. Majority are branch retinal vein compared to central retinal vein.
Signs/symptoms: Acute uniocular visual loss which is painless.
Diagnosis: Clinical examination and slit lamp examination/fundoscopy.
Risk factors: Hypertension, hyperlipidaemia, obesity, diabetes, glaucoma, chronic inflammation, anticardiolipin antibodies and hyperhomocysteinemia associated with retinal vein thrombosis.
Tx at diagnosis? Yes, future risk of recurrence around 10–15%.
First line tx: LMWH for 1–6 months depending on risk factors, warfarin, DOACS or anti-platelet **NOT** recommended.

Upper Extremity DVT

Epidemiology: 15:100,00 population and 10% of all DVT.
Signs/symptoms: Pain, swelling, CVC line not bloodletting, erythema. Diagnosed by USS doppler as per lower limb DVT.
Risk factors: CVC, thoracic outlet syndrome, trauma, malignancy, thrombophilia, surgery or limb immobilisation.
Tx at diagnosis? Yes.
First line tx: LMWH then warfarin or DOACS for 3–6 months. Surgical decompression in thoracic outlet syndrome.

Vena Cava Thrombosis

Epidemiology: Malignancy commonest cause of SVC DVT diagnosed on CT. IVC commonly affects intrarenal section and more common in women.
Signs/symptoms: Head and neck swelling, vein engorgement, SOB.
Diagnosis: CT Angio or CTPA.
If proximal DVT on doppler to image iliac veins and IVC.
Risk factors: Malignancy, CVC, infection, compression, IVC filter, lupus anticoagulant.
Tx at diagnosis? Yes, consider surgery in those with non-malignant causes and severe symptoms.
First line tx: LMWH initially and then warfarin or DOACS for 3–6 months. Consider catheter directed thrombolysis in acute severe IVC thrombosis.

Abdominal Vein Thrombosis. Includes Portal, Hepatic, Mesenteric and Splenic

Epidemiology: Relatively rare thrombosis commonly leading caused by underlying splenic or hepatic pathology.
Signs/symptoms: Abdominal pain, ascites, deranged liver function tests, splenic infarcts, bleeding.
Diagnosis: USS doppler as good as MRI or CT.
Risk factors: Cirrhosis, infection, MPN, trauma, PNH, APS, hepatomegaly, Budd-Chiari syndrome, bowel ischaemia, malignancy. Consider PNH screen in VTE at unusual site especially abdominal vein.
Tx at diagnosis? If cirrhosis be careful as high bleeding risk, otherwise yes. Involve gastro as part of MDT for decision making on bleeding vs thrombotic risk.
First line tx: LMWH or other long-term anticoagulation for 3–6 months or long term if MPN or APS. TIPSS procedure considered in those not for anticoagulation. DOACS can be considered after initial heparin treatment.

Ovarian Vein Thrombosis

Epidemiology: Occurs in 1:1,000 pregnancies.
Signs/symptoms: Abdominal pain, tachycardia, fever. Vague symptomatology. May embolise to PE.
Diagnosis: CT or MRI.
Risk factors: Complicated pregnancy, PID, recent surgery, infection.
Tx at diagnosis? Yes.
First line tx: LMWH or other anticoagulation for 3–6 months.

Superficial Vein Thrombosis of Lower Limb

Epidemiology: More common than DVT, commonly in females and in those with pre-existing varicose vein.

Signs/symptoms: Same as DVT.

Risk factors: Same as DVT. 10% progress to DVT within 1–2 weeks so follow up USS recommended.

Diagnosis: USS doppler.

Tx at diagnosis? No, depends on proximity to sapheno-femoral junction.

First line tx: Within 3 cm to sapheno-femoral junction treat with therapeutic anti-coagulation. If risk factors for extension to DVT or recurrence give prophylactic LMWH for 30 days or can now consider rivaroxaban. Everyone else NSAID for 1–2 weeks.

Guidelines:
https://onlinelibrary.wiley.com/doi/full/10.1111/j.1365-2141.2012.09249.x
https://onlinelibrary.wiley.com/doi/full/10.1111/bjh.18189

Cancer Associated VTE

Epidemiology: 10–20% of cancer patients will suffer a VTE and 20% of total VTE are cancer associated.

Signs/symptoms/diagnosis: As for VTE though may be harder to diagnose if SOB already from treatment or disease.

Risk factors:

Cancer related: High WCC in leukaemia, monoblastic AML, metastatic disease, certain tumours are more thrombotic than others.

Treatment related: CVC line, asparaginase therapy, surgery.

Other: Chemotherapy, immobility, dehydration, sepsis.

Tx at diagnosis? Yes, careful to consider bleeding risk and drug interactions as well as duration.

First line tx: Use of LMWH, warfarin and now DOACS all used.

Prophylaxis: With LMWH for all hospital in patients after assessing bleeding risk. TEDS in those where contraindicated.

Initial treatment: LMWH or DOACS and recommendations now from ASH are for DOACS over LMWH or warfarin going forward except for high bleeding risk tumour e.g., intra-luminal gastrointestinal.

Long term: Continue in those with active cancer or recurrent VTE. Often continue anti-coagulation until 3 months post treatment and in remission unless increased bleeding risk. DOACS or LMWH recommended for > 6 months. Often minimum treatment for cancer associated VTE 6 months.

Monitoring: As for VTE.

Trials to quote: NEJM trial: Apixaban vs LMWH in cancer VTE non-inferior and no increased bleeding risk.

Other considerations: Platelet monitoring during chemo, hold treatment dose if < 50 and prophylaxis if < 30. Consider IVC filter or split dose in this scenario. If hospital inpatient and high risk (< 4 weeks since thrombosis) consider UFH infusion and anti-Xa monitoring. Consider whether DOACS appropriate based on cancer type i.e., GI or GU cancers which have higher bleeding risk on DOACS.

Guidelines:

https://ashpublications.org/bloodadvances/article/5/4/927/475194/American-Society-of-Hematology-2021-guidelines-for

https://www.thelancet.com/journals/lanonc/article/PIIS1470-2045(22)00160-7/fulltext

Inherited Thrombophilia

Introduction: Inherited thrombophilia are characterised by mutations to factor V Leiden, protein C and S, prothrombin, antithrombin as well as others. I shall only discuss the above in this section and the risk they pose to thrombosis development.

Epidemiology: Varying incidence. Account for < 10% of recurrent VTE.

Population affected: Most thrombophilia are not recommended to be tested for at diagnosis of a VTE unless a relevant family history or other reason to suggest i.e., skin necrosis on warfarin then test protein C and S. Prevalence of mutation below.

AT: 0.02–0.2%.

PC/S deficiency: 0.5%.

Activated Protein C resistance: 5%.

Prothrombin: 2%.

FVL: 5%.

Signs/symptoms: As for VTE though some symptoms with certain thrombophilia, such as autoimmune link in APS. Purpura fulminans in neonates, screen for protein C and S deficiency.

Diagnosis: Molecular testing of the identified thrombophilia defect to see if homo/ heterozygous and the variant identified. Testing should be offered to a patient with VTE and a first degree relative with known thrombophilia where the result may alter treatment decisions or lifestyle. APS screen for in pregnancy associated VTE or recurrent miscarriage.

Tx at diagnosis? Yes, if associated with VTE. May change treatment in those with VTE and thrombophilia in certain high-risk scenarios i.e., during pregnancy.

Other important work up: Family history, still investigate for other provoking factors i.e., malignancy or APS. Perform APS screen after 3 months on anticoagulation so not to get false +ve results.

First line tx: Mostly the same as for VTE including time of treatment though most may want to stay on long term anticoagulation if thrombophilia despite relative risk mentioned below. In protein C or S deficiency do not generally use warfarin. If unusual site, follow guidance above.

Trials to quote: TIPPS: Thrombophilia in pregnancy prophylaxis study assessing LMWH prophylaxis in VTE prevention.

Guidelines:

https://onlinelibrary.wiley.com/doi/10.1111/bjh.18239

Antiphospholipid Syndrome

Incidence: Acquired autoimmune disorder characterised by thrombosis, pregnancy complications and specific antibody positivity.

Signs/symptoms: Recurrent VTE and unusual site, recurrent early (< 10/40) miscarriage, stillbirth or preterm labour, IUGR, pre-eclampsia, placental abruption, autoimmune symptoms, association with syndrome like SLE, livedo reticularis or nephrotic syndromes. May also be thrombocytopaenia. Prolonged APTT if lupus sensitive reagents used.

Diagnosis: At least 1 from lab and clinical criteria to make diagnosis.

Lab:

- LA, ACL or AB2GP1 present in medium or high titre on 2 occasions 12 weeks apart.

Clinical:

- VTE.
- 1 or more unexplained death of normal fetus after 10 weeks or preterm birth (< 34 weeks) due to eclampsia or placenta issue.
- 3 or more unexplained consecutive miscarriages before 10 weeks without other cause.

Testing: Prolonged phospholipid assays i.e., APTT. Presence of an inhibitor. Demonstrating that the inhibitor is phospholipid dependent. Use DRVVT and another assay for LA detection and confirmation with phospholipid dependent step. ELISA for antibodies. ACL and AB2GP1 can be done on anticoagulation. LA must be done off anticoagulation. Need to show persistence of antibodies at least 12 weeks apart.

When to test: Unprovoked proximal DVT or PE, stroke < 50-years-old, above clinical criteria related to pregnancy, recurrent VTE, VTE and family history of APS.

Tx at diagnosis? Yes, if diagnosed with VTE or other clinical criteria. No clinical criteria and incidental antibody positivity then no treatment or prophylaxis needed. May consider prophylaxis in pregnancy based on other associated risk factors.

Other important work up: Screen for autoimmune conditions, consider other thrombophilia, consider other provoking factors.

First line tx: Long-term anticoagulation advised. Warfarin in arterial and high risk i.e., triple +ve antibodies. DOACS can be given in non-arterial and non-triple +ve in certain scenarios but risk of arterial events shown to be higher on DOACS even if VTE was initial event so warfarin remains the mainstay of treatment for all; LMWH and Aspirin in pregnancy.

Specific scenarios:

Stroke: Warfarin and antiplatelet if high risk.

Pregnancy: LMWH and aspirin prophylaxis in all and treatment dose if thrombosis or > 3 pregnancy losses or any other obstetric criteria i.e., all APS need LMWH in pregnancy and aspirin in some form.

Catastrophic APS: Treatment dose anticoagulation with LMWH or heparin infusion, steroids, plasma exchange and ITU.

Trials to quote: <u>Leiden Thrombophilia Study</u>: Increased first DVT risk associated with LA and AB2GP1 antibodies.

Other considerations: <u>Catastrophic APS</u>: Life threatening multi-organ failure, use of RCOG green top guidance for anticoagulation duration postpartum and involving obstetrics in decision making. Hydroxychloroquine also used in thrombotic APS to immunosuppress.

Guidelines:

https://onlinelibrary.wiley.com/doi/full/10.1111/j.1365-2141.2012.09037.x

https://onlinelibrary.wiley.com/doi/full/10.1111/bjh.16308

https://ashpublications.org/blood/article/126/11/1285/34367/How-I-treat-catastrophic-thrombotic-syndromes

Heparin Induced Thrombocytopaenia

Introduction: Acquired immune mediated thrombocytopaenia due to the development of IgG antibodies against PF4 receptors on platelets following exposure to heparin.

Epidemiology: Higher risk in UFH compared to LMWH, surgical patients and trauma or orthopaedic patients.

Signs/symptoms: Platelet count typically falls 5–10 days after starting heparin or on re-exposure to heparin within 100 days, > 50% fall, new thrombosis, skin lesion at injection site. 40–50% develop thrombosis.

Diagnosis: Platelet activation and antigen studies for diagnosis of HIT. PF4 ELISA commonly performed and based on the rise in optical density can interpret likelihood of HIT. Reversal of test with use of high dose heparin confers a diagnosis of HIT. Other studies like serotonin release assay are more specific but requires expert lab, not commonly done despite high sensitivity and specificity.

- Clinical and pathological diagnosis.
- 4T score as screening looks at onset, degree of fall, new thrombosis and alternative causes.

Pre-test probability risk based on score of <u>Low</u>: 0–3. <u>Intermediate</u>: 4–5. <u>High</u>: > 5.

Pathophysiology: Heparin exposure leads to a confirmational change of PF4 receptor on platelets which leads to antibody development against the heparin-PF4 complex. Upon binding of platelets are further activated through Fc receptors leading to thrombocytopaenia but the production of pro-coagulant factors such as thrombin. HIT should be considered a pro-thrombotic condition despite thrombocytopaenia.

Tx at diagnosis? Yes. Hold heparin if suspected and if thrombosis will need anti-coagulant switching.

Other important work up: Rule out infection, drugs, cardiopulmonary surgery, MDS pr bone marrow pathology, ITP, TTP or other causes.

First line tx: Sequence of events below for suspected HIT after 4T score.

1. Stop Heparin in intermediate or high risk.
2. Switch to full dose alternative anticoagulant such as danaparoid, argatroban or fondaparinux in high risk and consider in intermediate.
3. Monitoring of platelet count to ensure improvement as well as anti-Xa in fondaparinux, danaparoid and APTT in argatroban.
4. Long term treatment with warfarin for 3 months if thrombosis, longer if multiple thrombosis. If no thrombosis treat for 1 month only.

Specific scenarios:

<u>Pregnancy</u>: Rare, stop heparin if suspect or confirmed and switch to any of the above alternative except warfarin. Need to involve obstetrics and consider bleeding risks such as spinal or epidural as well as delivery and thrombotic complications postpartum.

Mechanism of action of anticoagulants:

Danaparoid: Direct Xa and thrombin inhibitor to a lesser degree, no effect on APTT or PT, half-life 24 hours.

Argatroban: Direct thrombin inhibitor, hepatic metabolism so use in renal dysfunction, can prolong PT.

Fondaparinux: Indirect Xa inhibitor by inhibition of antithrombin-III, half-life 16–20 hours.

Important side effects: Bleeding on anticoagulant, consider local measures if possible, i.e., compression or TXA washes.

Do not give platelets unless severe, life-threatening bleeding and even then, should be discussed with specialist.

Other considerations: Any heparin exposure should have baseline platelet count with more care and follow up in higher risk patients, patient alert card, plan for different VTE prophylaxis for future surgeries etc due to risk of repeat HIT if re-exposed.

Guidelines:

https://onlinelibrary.wiley.com/doi/full/10.1111/bjh.12059
https://practical-haemostasis.com/Miscellaneous/hit_assays.html

4T score.

Criteria	Score of 1	Score of 2	Total score	Risk and action
Thrombocytopaenia degree	30–50% fall or nadir 10–19×10^9/L	50% fall and nadir $\geq 20 \times 10^9$/L	≤ 3	Low: Monitor
Timing of fall	Likely 5–10 days post-exposure, ≤ 1 day or > 10 day with exposure to heparin within 30–100 days	Clearly 5–10 days postexposure or ≤ 1 day with exposure to heparin within 30 days	4–5	Intermediate: Send PF4 antibodies and consider switch of heparin product
Thrombosis	Progressive or recurrent thrombosis or new suspected.	Confirmed or skin necrosis or acute reaction after IV heparin bolus	≥ 6	High: Send PF4 antibodies and switch heparin product
Other cause for Thrombocytopaenia	Possible	None		

Vaccine-induced Immune Thrombocytopaenia and Thrombosis

Introduction: VITT is a rare complication following COVID-19 vaccination leading to mild to severe thrombocytopaenia with associated thrombosis and +ve PF4 antibodies. Untreated the mortality is high. Thrombosis can occur at any site, including and often cerebral or atypical sites such as splanchnic vein.

Incidence: 50% mortality if left untreated. Incidence around 1:100,000 with no sex predominance. More reported cases with AstraZeneca and Johnson and Johnson vaccines than others.

Signs/symptoms: Headache or focal neurological signs, local symptoms of thrombosis i.e., calf swelling, bleeding or petechial rash, ICB, fever, myalgia, lethargy. All following vaccination.

Bloods: Thrombocytopaenia, D-dimer elevated, hypofibrinogenemia, +ve PF4 antibodies by ELISA, associated organ dysfunction from clot i.e., liver dysfunction in abdominal vein thrombosis.

Diagnosis: Meet all 5 criteria below.
- COVID-19 vaccine within 4–42 days of symptoms starting.
- Thrombocytopaenia.
- +ve PF4 antibodies.
- D-dimer 4 × ULN.
- New confirmed arterial or venous thrombosis via imaging.

Pathophysiology: Not dissimilar to HIT. Following vaccination PF4 antibodies are produced in the absence of heparin against the vaccine and lead to platelet activation and consumption causing thrombocytopaenia. Activation leads to vessel wall adhesion and activation of the coagulation cascade and prothrombotic complexes leading to VTE formation.

Tx at diagnosis? Yes. Treat if new thrombosis, vaccine history and thrombocytopaenia +/- elevated D-dimer × 4 ULN. If no thrombosis, vaccine history, symptoms and raised D-dimer and low fibrinogen then send PF4 and rescan. If PF4 is -ve then the chance of being VITT is incredibly low and should consider other conditions such as ITP.

Other important work up: Drug history, virology or infection screen for other causes of thrombocytopaenia, blood film, autoimmune screen.

First line tx: IVIG at a dose of 1 g/kg OD for 2 days. PLEX in severe or refractory disease. If refractory, consider rituximab and high dose steroids also though limited successful evidence. Anticoagulate with non-heparin product as per HIT once bleeding risk satisfactory i.e., DOACS fondaparinux or danaparoid. FGN replacement targeting > 1.5 g/L.

Important side effects: +ve hepatitis and TB serology following IVIG and steroid complications as previously mentioned.

Monitoring: Recheck D-dimer, platelets, FGN and PF4 antibodies weekly for 1 month then monthly for 6 months. Continue anticoagulation for 3 months minimum and can stop once normal D-dimer, platelets, FGN and -ve PF4 antibodies. Provide a patient information leaflet and patient alert card.

Other considerations: Avoid platelet transfusion at all costs unless severe life or limb threatening bleeding, discussion with coagulation specialist and transfer to tertiary centre, COVID-19 mortality in those unvaccinated and haematology patients higher than risk of VITT, consider other branded vaccinations such as Moderna in those with VITT or previous history of HIT. TXA or other adjuncts in bleeding, neurosurgical intervention in Cerebral sinus thrombosis with ICB, yellow card and inform haematology pharmacy, antiplatelet agent in arterial thrombosis after 1 month.

Guidelines:

https://b-s-h.org.uk/media/20499/guidance-version-22-20210903.pdf

https://www.hematology.org/covid-19/vaccine-induced-immune-thrombotic-thrombocytopenia

Essay Writing Technique

It's not a secret that essay writing isn't a brilliantly taught skill at medical school. Our postgraduate exams are often multiple choice, so we don't get many opportunities to develop our technique and hone this craft. Below are a few essay writing tips and some important buzzwords to add into your essays which help to demonstrate a holistic approach to the question you're asked.

1. Practice, practice, practice

It might sound obvious but starting to practise early is key. For me, not starting early enough was a mistake and the longer I left it the more of a "thing" it became. To get going, pick a subject you enjoy and start writing an essay. Simple as that. Not a literature review by any means but start with something like a 200-word essay on different treatments in AML. Alternatively, you could write a letter to the editor of a journal; it's a great way to focus your writing and it might result in a publication! Once you've done your first small essay, you'll see it's not so daunting and from there, you'll be flying!

2. Time yourself

This again sounds obvious but not everyone does it. It's no good writing a perfectly crafted essay on neonatal transfusion requirements if you take 2 hours to finish it. The guidance is to allow 45 minutes for each domain of the exam with 2–3 questions in each. This question with the highest weighting will be the essay you should spend most time on as it's the bulk of the marks. Plan your essay at the beginning of the time with headings, sections and bullet points, and build it from there.

3. Have someone mark your essay

I would say this is probably the most useful advice I can give you. Nearly all your consultants have done this exam and now set questions for it or act as examiners. They can tell you what makes a good read and what things don't sound good or even annoy them when marking. They can give you clarity on what is the best way to formulate answers and get points across. As well as this, they can give you individual feedback on your writing style. I've found that most of them are very happy to help and they can be a really good resource.

4. Use experts to guide revision and uncover blind spots

Carrying on from above, use the advice they give you to develop your learning and not take it personally. If you get a rubbish mark from a consultant colleague on a mock essay, use it to build on and revisit your learning. It's much more useful for passing the exam getting a bad mark and correcting it with additional work than getting positive feedback all the time. You'll learn more from your mistakes than from your success.

5. Past papers

Use them! As well as the ones on the FRCPath website from previous exams there are numerous websites and paper banks with mock exams. Some particularly helpful consultant colleagues in my exam even set questions for a group of us each week and then marked them. Dr Fiona Regan, absolute legend.

6. Key phrases

Below are some buzzwords and key phrases you can add into your essay to help to round it off.

Clinical trial: Always consider especially in those who have relapsed or failed treatment.

MDT approach: This shows you have considered the wider picture and aren't thinking alone.

Escalate to seniors: Even though you may feel very confident managing a certain disorder it's important to be aware of your limitations and when you would escalate appropriately or make your consultant aware of a certain scenario i.e., new TTP.

CNS: The mention of a clinical nurse specialist shows you understand that these often new and life changing disorders come with questions and logistical steps that need to be planned and coordinated, like outpatient and day care appointments.

Late effects: Very important not to forget, especially in malignant haematology. 1 or 2 is sufficient and generally "secondary cancers later in life" covers most chemotherapies.

Palliative care: Often overlooked in essays but mentioning it as part of treatment lines and management plans is a good holistic approach.

Empowering the patient: Examiners love this. Using things like antibody/neutropaenic sepsis/irradiated blood component cards shows that you're not only empowering the patient but you're thinking about patient safety.

Registries: Mention in conditions like bleeding disorders i.e., VWD or ITP.

Acknowledgments

A massive thank you to all the consultants who have helped me to compile and review this book. John, Mamta, Caroline, Richard and Akila I really cannot thank you enough. My colleagues through the years who have helped give me ideas for the book as well as supported me in preparing for the exam and as a new haematology registrar. To mention a few: Chira Mustafa, Amita Ranger, Charlotte Wilding, Christina Crossette-Thambiah, Andy Hastings and George Adams. My best friend Charlie who reviewed the content (Charlie Butler Content) and edited the book. My friend Becky Mitchell for helping design the artwork (my own happy neutrophil!). My family and friends for always standing by me, understanding and never complaining that sometimes work crosses over into our personal lives. And finally, to all the patients and their loved ones that I have met in my time as a haematologist who bring me such fulfilment in my job and who I will always do my best for.

References

1. Sickle Cell Society (2018). *Standards for the clinical care of adults with sickle cell disease in the UK.* London: Sickle Cell Society.

2. www.nice.org.uk (2023). *Project information | Voxelotor for treating sickle cell disease [ID1403] | Guidance | NICE.* [online] Available at: https://www.nice.org.uk/guidance/indevelopment/gid-ta10505 [Accessed 27 Jul. 2023].

3. Frangoul, H., Altshuler, D., Cappellini, M.D., Chen, Y.-S., Domm, J., Eustace, B.K., Foell, J., de la Fuente, J., Grupp, S., Handgretinger, R., Ho, T.W., Kattamis, A., Kernytsky, A., Lekstrom-Himes, J., Li, A.M., Locatelli, F., Mapara, M.Y., de Montalembert, M., Rondelli, D. and Sharma, A. (2020). CRISPR-Cas9 Gene Editing for Sickle Cell Disease and β-Thalassemia. *New England Journal of Medicine,* [online] 384(3). doi:https://doi.org/10.1056/nejmoa2031054.

4. Provan, D., Baglin, T.P., Inderjeet Dokal and Johannes De Vos (2015). *Oxford handbook of clinical haematology.* Oxford: Oxford University Press.

5. LearnHaem (n.d.). *Haemoglobin SC Disease.* [online] LearnHaem | Haematology Made Simple. Available at: https://www.learnhaem.com/courses/frcpath-morph/lessons/thal-haemoglobinopathies/topic/sc-disease/#:~:text=Haemoglobin%20SC%20disease%20is%20a [Accessed 27 Jul. 2023].

6. NICE (2021). *Sickle cell disease: How common is sickle cell disease?* [online] NICE. Available at: https://cks.nice.org.uk/topics/sickle-cell-disease/background-information/prevalence/ [Accessed 27 Jul. 2023].

7. Centers for Disease Control and Prevention (2017). *What is Sickle Cell Trait?* [online] Centers for Disease Control and Prevention. Available at: https://www.cdc.gov/ncbddd/sicklecell/traits.html.

8. El Ariss AB, Younes M, Matar J, Berjaoui Z. Prevalence of Sickle Cell Trait in the Southern Suburb of Beirut, Lebanon. Mediterr J Hematol Infect Dis. 2016 Feb 20; 8(1):e2016015. doi: 10.4084/MJHID.2016.015. PMID: 26977274; PMCID: PMC4771139.

9. Gibson JS, Rees DC. How benign is sickle cell trait? EBioMedicine. 2016 Sep; 11:21-22. doi: 10.1016/j.ebiom.2016.08.023. Epub 2016 Aug 21. PMID: 27580691; PMCID: PMC5049987.

10. Soudabeh Hosseeini, Ebrahim Kalantari, Akbar Dorgalaleh, Taregh Bamedi, Massomeh Farzi, Dorgalele Saeed; Thalassemia and Hemoglobinopathy Screening By HPLC Method and Comparison With Conventional Methods. *Blood* 2013; 122 (21): 4709. doi: https://doi.org/10.1182/blood.V122.21.4709.4709.

11. George E, Jamal AR, Khalid F, Osman KA. High performance liquid chromatography (HPLC) as a screening tool for classical Beta-thalassaemia trait in malaysia. Malays J Med Sci. 2001 Jul; 8(2):40-6. PMID: 22893759; PMCID: PMC3413648.

12. Challenge TDT (n.d.). *Beta-Thalassemia Prevalence, Pathophysiology and Inheritance.* [online] Available at: https://www.challengetdt.com/genetics-and-pathophysiology [Accessed 27 Jul. 2023].

13. Daniel David Mais, MD and others, The Range of Hemoglobin A$_2$ in Hemoglobin E Heterozygotes as Determined by Capillary Electrophoresis, *American Journal of Clinical Pathology*, Volume 132, Issue 1, July 2009, pp. 34–38, https://doi.org/10.1309/AJCPP5OJIXXZVLSS.

14. Shanthala Devi AM, Rameshkumar K, Sitalakshmi S. Hb D: A Not So Rare Hemoglobinopathy. Indian J Hematol Blood Transfus. 2016 Jun; 32(Suppl 1):294-8. doi: 10.1007/s12288-013-0319-3. Epub 2014 Jan 22. PMID: 27408416; PMCID: PMC4925467.

15. Jomoui W, Fucharoen G, Sanchaisuriya K, Nguyen VH, Fucharoen S. Hemoglobin Constant Spring among Southeast Asian Populations: Haplotypic Heterogeneities and Phylogenetic Analysis. PLoS One. 2015 Dec 18; 10(12):e0145230. doi: 10.1371/journal.pone.0145230. PMID: 26683994; PMCID: PMC4686174.

16. Adams, R.J., McKie, V.C., Brambilla, D., Carl, E., Gallagher, D., Nichols, F.T., Roach, S., Abboud, M., Berman, B., Driscoll, C., Files, B., Hsu, L., Hurlet, A., Miller, S., Olivieri, N., Pegelow, C., Scher, C., Vichinsky, E., Wang, W. and Woods, G. (1998). Stroke Prevention Trial in Sickle Cell Anemia. *Controlled Clinical Trials*, 19(1), pp. 110–129. doi:https://doi.org/10.1016/s0197-2456(97)00099-8.

17. Margaret T. Lee, Sergio Piomelli, Suzanne Granger, Scott T. Miller, Shannon Harkness, Donald J. Brambilla, Robert J. Adams, for the STOP Study Investigators; Stroke Prevention Trial in Sickle Cell Anemia (STOP): extended follow-up and final results. *Blood* 2006; 108 (3): 847–852. doi: https://doi.org/10.1182/blood-2005-10-009506.

18. clinicaltrials.gov (n.d.). *Stroke Prevention in Sickle Cell Anemia (STOP 2) - Full Text View - ClinicalTrials.gov*. [online] Available at: https://classic.clinicaltrials.gov/ct2/show/NCT00006182 [Accessed 27 Jul. 2023].

19. Adams RJ, Brambilla D; Optimizing Primary Stroke Prevention in Sickle Cell Anemia (STOP 2) Trial Investigators. Discontinuing prophylactic transfusions used to prevent stroke in sickle cell disease. N Engl J Med. 2005 Dec 29; 353(26):2769-78. doi: 10.1056/NEJMoa050460. PMID: 16382063.

20. Ware RE *et al.*, Hydroxycarbamide versus chronic transfusion for maintenance of transcranial doppler flow velocities in children with sickle cell anaemia-TCD With Transfusions Changing to Hydroxyurea (TWiTCH): a multicentre, open-label, phase 3, non-inferiority trial. Lancet. 2016 Feb 13; 387(10019):661-670. doi: 10.1016/S0140-6736(15)01041-7. Epub 2015 Dec 6. PMID: 26670617; PMCID: PMC5724392.

21. Ware RE, Helms RW; SWiTCH Investigators. Stroke With Transfusions Changing to Hydroxyurea (SWiTCH). Blood. 2012 Apr 26; 119(17):3925-32. doi: 10.1182/blood-2011-11-392340. Epub 2012 Feb 7. PMID: 22318199; PMCID: PMC3350359.

22.   Frangoul, H., Altshuler, D., Cappellini, M.D., Chen, Y.-S., Domm, J., Eustace, B.K., Foell, J., de la Fuente, J., Grupp, S., Handgretinger, R., Ho, T.W., Kattamis, A., Kernytsky, A., Lekstrom-Himes, J., Li, A.M., Locatelli, F., Mapara, M.Y., de Montalembert, M., Rondelli, D. and Sharma, A. (2020). CRISPR-Cas9 Gene Editing for Sickle Cell Disease and β-Thalassemia. *New England Journal of Medicine*, [online] 384(3). doi:https://doi.org/10.1056/nejmoa2031054.

23.   Wang, W.C., Ware, R.E., Miller, S.T., Iyer, R.V., Casella, J.F., Minniti, C.P., Rana, S., Thornburg, C.D., Rogers, Z.R., Kalpatthi, R.V., Barredo, J.C., Brown, R.C., Sarnaik, S.A., Howard, T.H., Wynn, L.W., Kutlar, A., Armstrong, F.D., Files, B.A., Goldsmith, J.C. and Waclawiw, M.A. (2011). Hydroxycarbamide in very young children with sickle-cell anaemia: a multicentre, randomised, controlled trial (BABY HUG). *The Lancet*, 377(9778), pp. 1663–1672. doi:https://doi.org/10.1016/s0140-6736(11)60355-3.

24.   Warner, M.J. and Kamran, M.T. (2022). *Iron deficiency anemia*. [online] Nih.gov. Available at: https://www.ncbi.nlm.nih.gov/books/NBK448065/.

25.   Barcellini W. New Insights in the Pathogenesis of Autoimmune Hemolytic Anemia. Transfus Med Hemother. 2015 Sep; 42(5):287-93. doi: 10.1159/000439002. Epub 2015 Sep 7. PMID: 26696796; PMCID: PMC4678320.

26.   Roy, NB, Da Costa, L, Russo, R, Bianchi, P, Mañú-Pereira, MdM, Fermo, E, *et al.*, The use of next-generation sequencing in the diagnosis of rare inherited anaemias: A Joint BSH/EHA Good Practice Paper. *Br J Haematol.* 2022; 198: 459–477. https://doi.org/10.1111/bjh.18191.

27.   Achille Iolascon, Immacolata Andolfo, Roberta Russo; Congenital dyserythropoietic anemias. *Blood* 2020; 136 (11): 1274–1283.
      doi: https://doi.org/10.1182/blood.2019000948.

28.   NORD (National Organization for Rare Disorders) (2019). *Pyruvate Kinase Deficiency - NORD (National Organization for Rare Disorders)*. [online] Available at: https://rarediseases.org/rare-diseases/pyruvate-kinase-deficiency/.

29.   medlineplus.gov (n.d.). *Hereditary spherocytosis: MedlinePlus Genetics*. [online] Available at:
      https://medlineplus.gov/genetics/condition/hereditary-spherocytosis/#:~:text=Hereditary%20spherocytosis%20occurs%20in%201.

30.   Lavinya, A.A., Razali, R.A., Razak, M.A., Mohamed, R., Moses, E.J., Soundararajan, M., Bruce, L.J., Eswaran, J. and Yusoff, N.M. (2021). Homozygous Southeast Asian ovalocytosis in five live-born neonates. *Haematologica*, [online] 106(6), pp. 1758–1761. doi:https://doi.org/10.3324/haematol.2020.268581.

31.   rarediseases.info.nih.gov (n.d.). *Hereditary elliptocytosis | Genetic and Rare Diseases Information Center (GARD) – an NCATS Program*. [online] Available at: https://rarediseases.info.nih.gov/diseases/6621/hereditary-elliptocytosis.

32.   Grosse SD, Gurrin LC, Bertalli NA, Allen KJ. Clinical penetrance in hereditary hemochromatosis: estimates of the cumulative incidence of severe liver disease among HFE C282Y homozygotes. Genet Med. 2018 Apr; 20(4):383-389. doi: 10.1038/gim.2017.121. Epub 2017 Aug 3. PMID: 28771247; PMCID: PMC5797490.

33. Adams, P.C., Reboussin, D.M., Barton, J.C., McLaren, C.E., Eckfeldt, J.H., McLaren, G.D., Dawkins, F.W., Acton, R.T., Harris, E.L., Gordeuk, V.R., Leiendecker-Foster, C., Speechley, M., Snively, B.M., Holup, J.L., Thomson, E. and Sholinsky, P. (2005). Hemochromatosis and Iron-Overload Screening in a Racially Diverse Population. *New England Journal of Medicine*, 352(17), pp. 1769–1778. doi:https://doi.org/10.1056/nejmoa041534.

34. Hill, Q.A., Grainger, J.D., Thachil, J., Provan, D., Evans, G., Garg, M., Bradbury, C., Bagot, C., Kanis, J.A. and Compston, J.E. (2019). The prevention of glucocorticoid-induced osteoporosis in patients with immune thrombocytopenia receiving steroids: a British Society for Haematology Good Practice Paper. *British Journal of Haematology*, 185(3), pp. 410–417. doi:https://doi.org/10.1111/bjh.15735.

35. Cooper, N. (2017). State of the art - how I manage immune thrombocytopenia. *British Journal of Haematology*, 177(1), pp. 39–54. doi:https://doi.org/10.1111/bjh.14515.

36. Pavord S, Thachil J, Hunt BJ, Murphy M, Lowe G, Laffan M, Makris M, Newland AC, Provan D, Grainger JD, Hill QA. Practical guidance for the management of adults with immune thrombocytopenia during the COVID-19 pandemic. Br J Haematol. 2020 Jun; 189(6):1038-1043. doi: 10.1111/bjh.16775. Epub 2020 Jun 2. PMID: 32374026; PMCID: PMC7267627.

37. Ali MA, Anwar MY, Aiman W, Dhanesar G, Omar Z, Hamza M, Zafar M, Rengarajan HK, Maroules M. Safety and Efficacy of Tyrosine Kinase Inhibitors in Immune Thrombocytopenic Purpura: A Systematic Review of Clinical Trials. J Xenobiot. 2023 Jan 28; 13(1):29-41. doi: 10.3390/jox13010005. PMID: 36810430; PMCID: PMC9944448.

38. Jalbert, J.J., Chaudhari, U., Zhang, H., Weyne, J. and Shammo, J.M. (2019). Epidemiology of PNH and Real-World Treatment Patterns Following an Incident PNH Diagnosis in the US. *Blood*, 134(Supplement_1), pp. 3407–3407. doi:https://doi.org/10.1182/blood-2019-125867.

39. Brodsky, R.A. (2021). How I treat paroxysmal nocturnal hemoglobinuria. *Blood*, 137(10), pp. 1304–1309. doi:https://doi.org/10.1182/blood.2019003812.

40. Parker, C.J. (2016). Update on the diagnosis and management of paroxysmal nocturnal hemoglobinuria. *Hematology*, 2016(1), pp. 208–216. doi:https://doi.org/10.1182/asheducation-2016.1.208.

41. Socié G, Mary JY, de Gramont A, Rio B, Leporrier M, Rose C, Heudier P, Rochant H, Cahn JY, Gluckman E. Paroxysmal nocturnal haemoglobinuria: long-term follow-up and prognostic factors. French Society of Haematology. Lancet. 1996 Aug 31; 348(9027):573-7. doi: 10.1016/s0140-6736(95)12360-1. PMID: 8774569.

42. https://www.NationalInstituteforHealthandCareExcellence (n.d.). *BNF is only available in the UK*. [online] NICE. Available at: https://bnf.nice.org.uk/drugs/caplacizumab/ [Accessed 27 Jul. 2023].

43. www.nice.org.uk (2020). *Overview | Caplacizumab with plasma exchange and immunosuppression for treating acute acquired thrombotic thrombocytopenic purpura | Guidance | NICE*. [online] Available at: https://www.nice.org.uk/guidance/ta667 [Accessed 27 Jul. 2023].
44. Legendre, C.M., Licht, C., Muus, P., Greenbaum, L.A., Babu, S., Bedrosian, C., Bingham, C., Cohen, D.J., Delmas, Y., Douglas, K., Eitner, F., Feldkamp, T., Fouque, D., Furman, R.R., Gaber, O., Herthelius, M., Hourmant, M., Karpman, D., Lebranchu, Y. and Mariat, C. (2013). Terminal Complement Inhibitor Eculizumab in Atypical Hemolytic–Uremic Syndrome. *New England Journal of Medicine*, [online] 368(23), pp. 2169–2181. doi:https://doi.org/10.1056/nejmoa1208981.
45. Tubman, V.N. and Field, J.J. (2015). Sickle solubility test to screen for sickle cell trait: what's the harm? *Hematology*, 2015(1), pp. 433–435. doi:https://doi.org/10.1182/asheducation-2015.1.433.
46. medlineplus.gov (n.d.). *Hemoglobin Electrophoresis: MedlinePlus Medical Test*. [online] Available at: https://medlineplus.gov/lab-tests/hemoglobin-electrophoresis/#:~:text=Hemoglobin%20electrophoresis%20is%20a%20test.
47. Anon (2020). *Hemoglobin: Part 2 - Hemoglobin Electrophoresis, (Hb electro-phoresis) - Labpedia.net*. [online] Available at: https://labpedia.net/haemoglobin-electrophoresis-hb-electrophoresis/.
48. Lybrate (n.d.). *Heinz Bodies Blood Test - Test Results, Normal Range, Cost And More*. [online] Available at: https://www.lybrate.com/lab-test/heinz-bodies-blood [Accessed 27 Jul. 2023].
49. Huber, S., Baer, C., Hutter, S. *et al.*, AML classification in the year 2023: How to avoid a Babylonian confusion of languages. *Leukemia* **37**, 1413–1420 (2023). https://doi.org/10.1038/s41375-023-01909-w.
50. www.nice.org.uk (2023). *Overview | Ibrutinib with venetoclax for untreated chronic lymphocytic leukaemia | Guidance | NICE*. [online] Available at: https://www.nice.org.uk/guidance/ta891 [Accessed 10 Aug. 2023].
51. Bain, B.J., Bates, I., Laffan, M.A. and S Mitchell Lewis (2017). *Dacie and Lewis practical haematology*. Marrickville, Australia: Elsevier.
52. SEER (2018). *SEER Hematopoietic and Lymphoid Neoplasm Database*. [online] Available at: https://seer.cancer.gov/seertools/hemelymph/.
53. Leukaemia Foundation (n.d.). *Essential Thrombocythaemia (ET)*. [online] Available at: https://www.leukaemia.org.au/blood-cancer/myeloproliferative-neoplasms/essential-thrombocythaemia/.
54. Leukaemia Foundation (n.d.). *Polycythaemia (Rubra) Vera*. [online] Available at: https://www.leukaemia.org.au/blood-cancer/myeloproliferative-neoplasms/polycythaemia-rubra-vera/.

55. Moulard, O., Mehta, J., Olivares, R., Iqbal, U. and Mesa, R.A. (2012). Epidemiology of Myelofibrosis (MF), Polycythemia Vera (PV) and Essential Thrombocythemia (ET) in the European Union (EU). *Blood*, 120(21), pp. 1744–1744. doi:https://doi.org/10.1182/blood.v120.21.1744.1744.

56. Dispenzieri, A. (2012). How I treat POEMS syndrome. *Blood*, 119(24), pp. 5650–5658. doi:https://doi.org/10.1182/blood-2012-03-378992.

57. Cancer Research UK. (2015). *Myeloma survival statistics*. [online] Available at: https://www.cancerresearchuk.org/health-professional/cancer-statistics/statistics-by-cancer-type/myeloma/survival#heading-Zero.

58. Mina, R., Joseph, N.S., Kaufman, J.L., Gupta, V.A., Heffner, L.T., Hofmeister, C.C., Boise, L.H., Dhodapkar, M.V., Gleason, C., Nooka, A.K. and Lonial, S. (2018). Survival outcomes of patients with primary plasma cell leukemia (pPCL) treated with novel agents. *Cancer*, 125(3), pp. 416–423. doi:https://doi.org/10.1002/cncr.31718.

59. Alaggio R *et al.*, The 5th edition of the World Health Organization Classification of Haematolymphoid Tumours: Lymphoid Neoplasms. Leukemia. 2022 Jul; 36(7):1720-1748. doi: 10.1038/s41375-022-01620-2. Epub 2022 Jun 22. Erratum in: Leukemia. 2023 Sep; 37(9):1944-1951. PMID: 35732829; PMCID: PMC9214472.

60. www.mds-hub.com (n.d.). *International Consensus Classification of MDS: 2022 updates*. [online] Available at: https://mds-hub.com/medical-information/international-consensus-classification-of-mds-2022-updates [Accessed 27 Jul. 2023].

61. Daniel A. *et al.*, International Consensus Classification of Myeloid Neoplasms and Acute Leukemias: integrating morphologic, clinical, and genomic data. *Blood* 2022; 140 (11): 1200–1228. doi: https://doi.org/10.1182/blood.2022015850.

62. Hartmut Döhner, Andrew H. Wei, Frederick R. Appelbaum, Charles Craddock, Courtney D. DiNardo, Hervé Dombret, Benjamin L. Ebert, Pierre Fenaux, Lucy A. Godley, Robert P. Hasserjian, Richard A. Larson, Ross L. Levine, Yasushi Miyazaki, Dietger Niederwieser, Gert Ossenkoppele, Christoph Röllig, Jorge Sierra, Eytan M. Stein, Martin S. Tallman, Hwei-Fang Tien, Jianxiang Wang, Agnieszka Wierzbowska, Bob Löwenberg; Diagnosis and management of AML in adults: 2022 recommendations from an international expert panel on behalf of the ELN. *Blood* 2022; 140 (12): 1345–1377. doi: https://doi.org/10.1182/blood.2022016867.

63. Gaidano G, Rossi D. The mutational landscape of chronic lymphocytic leukemia and its impact on prognosis and treatment. Hematology Am Soc Hematol Educ Program. 2017 Dec 8; 2017(1):329-337. doi: 10.1182/asheducation-2017.1.329. PMID: 29222275; PMCID: PMC6142556.

64. Pardanani, A. (2018). Systemic mastocytosis in adults: 2019 update on diagnosis, risk stratification and management. *American Journal of Hematology*. doi:https://doi.org/10.1002/ajh.25371.

65. www.mll.com (n.d.). *The New WHO Classification 2022*. [online] Available at: https://www.mll.com/en/the-new-who-classification-2022.

66.   Alaggio R *et al.*, The 5th edition of the World Health Organization Classification of Haematolymphoid Tumours: Lymphoid Neoplasms. Leukemia. 2022 Jul; 36(7):1720-1748. doi: 10.1038/s41375-022-01620-2. Epub 2022 Jun 22. Erratum in: Leukemia. 2023 Jul 19; PMID: 35732829; PMCID: PMC9214472.

67.   Adams SV, Newcomb PA, Shustov AR. Racial Patterns of Peripheral T-Cell Lymphoma Incidence and Survival in the United States. J Clin Oncol. 2016 Mar 20; 34(9):963-71. doi: 10.1200/JCO.2015.63.5540. PMID: 26962200; PMCID: PMC5070555.

68.   Khoury, J.D., Solary, E., Abla, O. *et al.*, The 5th edition of the World Health Organization Classification of Haematolymphoid Tumours: Myeloid and Histiocytic/Dendritic Neoplasms. *Leukemia* **36**, 1703–1719 (2022). https://doi.org/10.1038/s41375-022-01613-1.

69.   www.mds-hub.com (n.d.). *International Consensus Classification of MDS: 2022 updates*. [online] Available at: https://mds-hub.com/medical-information/international-consensus-classification-of-mds-2022-updates [Accessed 27 Jul. 2023].

70.   NHS Blood and Transplant (2019). *Blood donation statistics*. [online] NHS Blood and Transplant. Available at: https://www.nhsbt.nhs.uk/how-you-can-help/get-involved/share-statistics/blood-donation-statistics/.

71.   NHS Blood Donation (2019). *Who can give blood*. [online] Available at: https://www.blood.co.uk/who-can-give-blood/.

72.   Guidelines for the Blood Transfusion Services (n.d.). Available at: https://www.transfusionguidelines.org/red-book/chapter-5-collection-of-a-blood-or-component-donation.pdf [Accessed 27 Jul. 2023].

73.   https://www.blood.co.uk/why-give-blood/blood-types/. Gehrie, E.A. and Tobian, A.A.R. (2020). PATCHing platelet data to improve transfusion. *Blood*, 135(16), pp. 1309–1310. doi:https://doi.org/10.1182/blood.2020005384.

74.   Caram-Deelder, C., Kreuger, A.L., Evers, D., de Vooght, K.M.K., van de Kerkhof, D., Visser, O., Péquériaux, N.C.V., Hudig, F., Zwaginga, J.J., van der Bom, J.G. and Middelburg, R.A. (2017). Association of Blood Transfusion From Female Donors With and Without a History of Pregnancy With Mortality Among Male and Female Transfusion Recipients. *JAMA*, [online] 318(15), pp. 1471–1478. doi:https://doi.org/10.1001/jama.2017.14825.

75.   www.reprocell.com (n.d.). *Protocol for buffy coat preparation from whole blood*. [online] Available at: https://www.reprocell.com/blog/biopta/buffy-coat-preparation-from-whole-blood [Accessed 21 Mar. 2023].

76.   Boulton, F.E. and James, V. (2007). Guidelines for policies on alternatives to allogeneic blood transfusion. 1. Predeposit autologous blood donation and transfusion. *Transfusion Medicine*, 17(5), pp. 354–365. doi:https://doi.org/10.1111/j.1365-3148.2007.00744.x.

77. Exchange therapy and continuous hemodiafiltration. CEN Case Rep. 2018 May; 7(1):114-120. doi: 10.1007/s13730-018-0307-4. Epub 2018 Jan 31. PMID: 29383577; PMCID: PMC5886938.

78. Serious Hazards of Transfusion (n.d.). *SHOT Annual Reports and Summaries*. [online] Available at: https://www.shotuk.org/shot-reports/ [Accessed 9 Mar. 2021].

79. Ma L, Danoff TM, Borish L: Case fatality and population mortality associated with anaphylaxis in the United States. J Allergy Clin Immunol 133 (4):1075–1083, 2014. doi: 10.1016/j.jaci.2013.10.029.

80. Soutar, R., McSporran, W., Tomlinson, T., Booth, C. and Grey, S. (2023). Guideline on the investigation and management of acute transfusion reactions. *British Journal of Haematology*. doi:https://doi.org/10.1111/bjh.18789.

81. Conti, F.M., Hitomi Yokoyama, A.P., Dezan, M.R., Costa, T.H., Aravechia, M.G., Mota, M.A. and Kutner, J.M. (2013). Diagnosis and Management Of POST-Transfusion Purpura - Case Report. *Blood*, 122(21), pp. 4834–4834. doi:https://doi.org/10.1182/blood.v122.21.4834.4834.

82. NICE (n.d.). *CKS is only available in the UK*. [online] Available at: https://cks.nice.org.uk/topics/hepatitis-c/.

83. CDC (2022). *Understanding the HIV Window Period | Testing | HIV Basics | HIV/AIDS | CDC*. [online] www.cdc.gov. Available at: https://www.cdc.gov/hiv/basics/hiv-testing/hiv-window-period.html.

84. CDC (2021). *Hepatitis B FAQs for Health Professionals | CDC*. [online] Centers for Disease Control and Prevention. Available at: https://www.cdc.gov/hepatitis/hbv/hbvfaq.htm#:~:text=primary%20liver%20cancer).-.

85. www.cdc.gov (2022). *Hepatitis C Questions and Answers for Health Professionals | CDC*. [online] Available at: https://www.cdc.gov/hepatitis/hcv/hcvfaq.htm#:~:text=People%20who%20have%20been%20very [Accessed 27 Jul. 2023].

86. wwwnc.cdc.gov (n.d.). *Hepatitis E | CDC Yellow Book 2024*. [online] Available at: https://wwwnc.cdc.gov/travel/yellowbook/2024/infections-diseases/hepatitis-e#:~:text=The%20incubation%20period%20of%20HEV [Accessed 27 Jul. 2023].

87. labtestsonline.org.uk (n.d.). *HTLV*. [online] Available at: https://labtestsonline.org.uk/tests/htlv#:~:text=The%20HTLV%20window%20period%20for [Accessed 27 Jul. 2023].

88. www.cdc.gov (2021). *Clinical and Pathologic Characteristics | Variant Creutzfeldt-Jakob Disease, Classic (CJD) | Prion Disease | CDC*. [online] Available at: https://www.cdc.gov/prions/vcjd/clinical-pathologic-characteristics.html/ [Accessed 27 Jul. 2023].

89. MAJOR OBSTETRIC HAEMORRHAGE (MOH) (This includes both antepartum and postpartum haemorrhage) Maternity Guideline (n.d.). Available at: https://smh-gas.org.uk/wp-content/uploads/2016/10/MOH.pdf [Accessed 27 Jul. 2023].

90. PAEDIATRIC MAJOR HAEMORRHAGE PROTOCOL (n.d.). Available at: https://smh-gas.org.uk/wp-content/uploads/2021/03/4.1.14-Paediatric-Major-Haemorrhage-Protocol-v8.4-1.pdf [Accessed 27 Jul. 2023].

91. Ltd, T.I.S. (n.d.). *JPAC - Transfusion Guidelines*. [online] transfusionguidelines.org. uk. Available at: https://www.transfusionguidelines.org/about [Accessed 27 Jul. 2023].

92. Mhra.gov.uk (2014). *Login*. [online] Available at: https://aic.mhra.gov.uk/mda/sabresystem.nsf/Login?Open [Accessed 27 Jul. 2023].

93. yellowcard.mhra.gov.uk (n.d.). *Blood factor and immunoglobulin products | Making medicines and medical devices safer*. [online] Available at: https://yellowcard.mhra.gov.uk/bloodfactors [Accessed 27 Jul. 2023].

94. UK NEQAS (2017). *Home - UK NEQAS | External Quality Assessment Services*. [online] Available at: https://ukneqas.org.uk/ [Accessed 27 Jul. 2023].

95. Hospitals and Science - NHSBT (n.d.). *Additional test implemented for Hepatitis B to identify donors with past Hep B*. [online] Available at: https://hospital.blood.co.uk/the-update/additional-test-implemented-for-hepatitis-b-to-identify-donors-with-past-hep-b/ [Accessed 10 Aug. 2023].

96. UKAS (n.d.). *About us*. [online] Available at: https://www.ukas.com/about-us/#:~:text=The%20United%20Kingdom%20Accreditation%20Service [Accessed 27 Jul. 2023].

97. Labpedia.net (2020). *Blood banking:- part 1- Blood Groups ABO and Rh System, Blood Grouping Procedures*. [online] Available at: https://labpedia.net/blood-banking-part-1-blood-groups-abo-and-rh-system-blood-grouping-procedures/ [Accessed 27 Jul. 2023].

98. LTG (2020). *ABO blood groups and Rh type Testing*. [online] Lab Tests Guide. Available at: https://www.labtestsguide.com/abo-grouping [Accessed 27 Jul. 2023].

99. Blood Bank Guy (2016). *Glossary: Antibody Screen - Blood Bank Guy Glossary*. [online] Available at: https://www.bbguy.org/education/glossary/gla20/ [Accessed 27 Jul. 2023].

100. Antibody Screening: Overview, Clinical Indications/Applications, Test Performance (2021). *eMedicine*. [online] Available at: https://emedicine.medscape.com/article/1731232-overview?icd=login_success_fb_match_norm&isSocialFTC=true#a1 [Accessed 27 Jul. 2023].

101. Dean, L. (2005). *Blood groups and red cell antigens*. Bethesda, Md.: NCBI.

102. Norfolk, D. and United Kingdom Blood Services (2013). *Handbook of transfusion medicine*. London: H.M.S.O.

103. Rish (2018). *The Lutheran blood group system*. [online] The Biomedical Scientist. Available at: https://thebiomedicalscientist.net/science/lutheran-blood-group-system?&redirectcounter=1 [Accessed 27 Jul. 2023].

104. Hellberg, Å. (2019). P1PK: a blood group system with an identity crisis. 15(1), pp. 40–45. doi:https://doi.org/10.1111/voxs.12505.

105. ADoung (2019). *The Lewis Blood Group System and Secretor Status.* [online] The Biomedical Scientist. Available at: https://thebiomedicalscientist.net/science/lewis-blood-group-system-and-secretor-status [Accessed 27 Jul. 2023].

106. Admin (2019). *Direct Coombs Test (DAT): Principle, Procedure, Interpretations and Confirmation.* [online] Medical Laboratory Scientist - MLS. Available at: https://medicallabscientist.org/direct-coombs-test-dat-principle-procedure-interpretations-and-confirmation/. [Accessed 27 Jul. 2023].

107. Zantek, N.D., Koepsell, S.A., Tharp, D.R. and Cohn, C.S. (2012). The direct antiglobulin test: A critical step in the evaluation of hemolysis. *American Journal of Hematology*, 87(7), pp. 707–709. doi:https://doi.org/10.1002/ajh.23218.

108. www.labce.com (n.d.). *PCH Donath-Landsteiner Test - LabCE.com, Laboratory Continuing Education.* [online] Available at: https://www.labce.com/spg670227_pch_donath_landsteiner_test.aspx.

109. Austin, E., Bates, S., De Silva, M., Howarth, D., Lubenko, A., Rowley, M., Scott, M., Thomas, E., White, J. and Williams, M. (2009). *Guidelines for the Estimation of Fetomaternal Haemorrhage Working Party of the British Committee for Standards in Haematology, Transfusion Taskforce. Writing group.* [online] Available at: https://b-s-h.org.uk/media/15705/transfusion-austin-the-estimation-of-fetomaternal-haemorrhage.pdf?cf=638034153929970000.

110. Black, L. (2013). *Bloody easy: coagulation simplified.* Toronto: Orbcon, Ontario Regional Blood Coordinating Network.

111. labtestsonline.org.uk (n.d.). aPTT. [online] Available at: https://labtestsonline.org.uk/tests/aptt#:~:text=A%20prolonged%20aPTT%20usually%20means [Accessed 27 Jul. 2023].

112. Tripodi, A., Chantarangkul, V., Martinelli, I., Bucciarelli, P. and Mannucci, P.M. (2004). A shortened activated partial thromboplastin time is associated with the risk of venous thromboembolism. *Blood*, 104(12), pp. 3631–3634. doi:https://doi.org/10.1182/blood-2004-03-1042.

113. Cleveland Clinic Labs. Background information (1995). *APMIS*, 103(S49), pp. 6–13. doi:https://doi.org/10.1111/j.1600-0463.1995.tb05528.x [Accessed 27 Jul. 2023].

114. www.pathologyoutlines.com (n.d.). *Mixing studies.* [online] Available at: https://www.pathologyoutlines.com/topic/coagulationmixingstudies.html [Accessed 27 Jul. 2023].

115. Synnovis (n.d.). *von Willebrand disease profile (VWF:RCo, VWF:Ag, VWF:CBA, FVIII).* [online] Available at: http://www.viapath.co.uk/our-tests/von-willebrand-disease-profile-vwfrco-vwfag-vwfcb-fviii [Accessed 27 Jul. 2023].

116. CDC (2020). *Data and Statistics on von Willebrand Disease | CDC*. [online] Centers for Disease Control and Prevention. Available at: https://www.cdc.gov/ncbddd/vwd/data.html#:~:text=Von%20Willebrand%20disease%20(VWD)%20occurs [Accessed 27 Jul. 2023].

117. Medlineplus.gov (n.d.). *Factor V Leiden thrombophilia: MedlinePlus Genetics*. [online] Available at: https://medlineplus.gov/genetics/condition/factor-v-leiden-thrombophilia/#:~:text=Factor%20V%20Leiden%20is%20the%20most%20common%20inherited%20form%20of [Accessed 27 Jul. 2023].

118. Anderson, F.A. (2003). Risk Factors for Venous Thromboembolism. *Circulation*, [online] 107(90231), pp. 9I–16. doi:https://doi.org/10.1161/01.cir.0000078469.07362.e6.

119. Perrier A, Desmarais S, Goehring C, de Moerloose P, Morabia A, Unger PF, Slosman D, Junod A, Bounameaux H. D-dimer testing for suspected pulmonary embolism in outpatients. Am J Respir Crit Care Med. 1997 Aug; 156(2 Pt 1):492-6. doi: 10.1164/ajrccm.156.2.9702032. PMID: 9279229.

120. Kirchmaier CM, Pillitteri D. Diagnosis and Management of Inherited Platelet Disorders. Transfus Med Hemother. 2010; 37(5):237-246. doi: 10.1159/000320257. Epub 2010 Sep 15. PMID: 21113246; PMCID: PMC2980508.

121. Harrison, P., Mackie, I., Mumford, A., Briggs, C., Liesner, R., Winter, M. and Machin, S. (2011). Guidelines for the laboratory investigation of heritable disorders of platelet function. B*ritish Journal of Haematology*, 155(1), pp. 30–44. doi:https://doi.org/10.1111/j.1365-2141.2011.08793.x.

122. Fahrni J, Husmann M, Gretener SB, Keo HH. Assessing the risk of recurrent venous thromboembolism--a practical approach. Vasc Health Risk Manag. 2015 Aug 17; 11:451-9. doi: 10.2147/VHRM.S83718. PMID: 26316770; PMCID: PMC4544622.

123. Kirchmaier CM, Pillitteri D. Diagnosis and Management of Inherited Platelet Disorders. Transfus Med Hemother. 2010; 37(5):237-246. doi: 10.1159/000320257. Epub 2010 Sep 15. PMID: 21113246; PMCID: PMC2980508.

124. Israels, S.J., Kahr, W.H.A., Blanchette, V.S., Luban, N.L.C., Rivard, G.E. and Rand, M.L. (2011). Platelet disorders in children: A diagnostic approach. *Pediatric Blood & Cancer*, 56(6), pp. 975–983. doi:https://doi.org/10.1002/pbc.22988.

Index

Printed in the USA
CPSIA information can be obtained
at www.ICGtesting.com
LVHW012031250824
789119LV00004B/15